# SPANISH TO GO
# For Medical Professionals

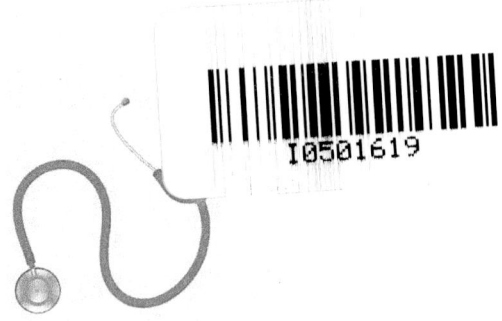

ONE STOP 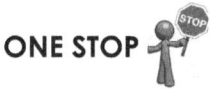 ENGLISH TO SPANISH REFERENCE

GUIDE

ENGLISH TO SPANISH MEDICAL VOCABULARY
ANATOMY SECTION
GRAMMAR SECTION
REFERENCE GUIDE

Written By:
Georgia Patilis
Illustrations by
Tina Pavlatos

Copyright © 2021 by Georgia Patilis

All rights reserved.

**IN LOVING MEMORY OF MY FATHER,
ANDREW PATILIS**

Dear Dad,

This book is dedicated to you, with my deepest love and respect for the selfless sacrifices that you made for your family.

You worked countless hours to make sure that your children would have the education and opportunities that were not availed to you.

Andrew Patilis, my dad, my hero. Not like the ones in the movies. A real life hero, who sacrificed his own dreams so that his children would have a better life. Your love for your family knew no bounds. Your family was your core and you led by love and example.

May you rest in peace in Heaven.

# TABLE OF CONTENTS

## Essential Doctor/Patient Vocabulary

Receptionist/Preliminary Patient Information ............... 2-4
Medical History (Illnesses) ............................................. 5-6
Doctor's Visit /Patient Information.................................. 7-8
Vital Signs ................................................................... 9-10

## Rx-Medications

    Types of Medications/Prescriptions........................... 11
    Units of Measure ....................................................... 12
    Storage of Medication ............................................... 12
    Prescription Label...................................................... 13
    Instructions for Taking Medication ...................... 14-15

## Hospital-Personnel/Tests/Equipment

X Rays & Tests................................................................ 16
THE HOSPITAL/MEDICAL PERSONNEL/
Emergency Professions & Equipment.......................... 17-19

## Pain

EXPRESSING PAIN: tener dolor vs doler ................ 20-23
WONG BAKER PAIN CHART ................................... 24
Pain Assessment & Types of Pain...................................... 25
Ailments/Symptoms ................................................. 26-27

## FIRST AID

    First Aid Kit .............................................................. 29
    First Aid Vocabulary ................................................. 30
    First Aid Code of Conduct & Procedures.................. 31
Heart Attack ................................................................... 32
Choking /Asphyxia ......................................................... 33
Burns .............................................................................. 34
Wounds .......................................................................... 35
Hemorrhages .................................................................. 36
Fractures ......................................................................... 37

**SPECIALTY CARE**
Cardiology ................................................................... 38–39
Endocrinology ........................................................... 40–41
Oncology ....................................................................... 42
Dental ...................................................................... 43–45
Eye ........................................................................... 46–47
Dermatology ............................................................ 48–50
ANATOMY ............................................................. 51–60
GRAMMAR ............................................................ 61–90
REFERENCE GUIDE .............................................. 91–95
WORKBOOK ....................................................... 96–173

# PART I

## ESSENTIAL DOCTOR / PATIENT VOCABULARY

# RECEPTIONIST / PRELIMINARY PATIENT INFORMATION DEL PACIENTE / RECEPCIONISTA / INFORMACION PRELIMINAR

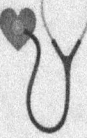

Receptionist/preliminary patient information,
Recepcionista/información preliminar del paciente

### Patient Demographics
What is your...? ¿Cuál es su...?

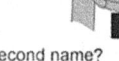

name, (first and last name), second name, nombre y apellido, second name?
¿Cómo se llama?
date of birth, fecha de nacimiento
social security number, número de seguro social
nationality/race, origen étnico /raza
primary language/preferred language, idioma primario, idioma preferido

What is your...?, ¿Cuál es su ...?
address /city/state/zip code, dirección/ciudad/estado/código postal
home telephone number, número de teléfono
cell number, número de teléfono celular
e-mail address, dirección de correo electrónico

### Civil Status/marital status, Estado civil
Are you.. ?, ¿Es Usted ....?
single, soltero,a
married, casado,a
separated, separado,a
divorced, divorciado,a
widow, widower, viudo, viuda
living together, viviendo juntos/unión libre

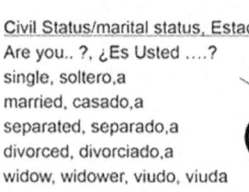
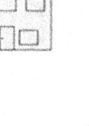

### Gender/Sexual Orientation, Género/orientación sexual
What is your gender?, ¿Cuál es su sexo?
male, masculino
female, femenino
What is your sexual orientation?, ¿Cuál es su orientación sexual?
heterosexual, heterosexual
homosexual, homosexual
bisexual, bisexualidad
transgender, transgénero

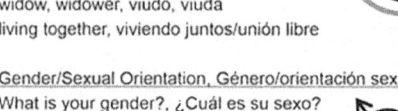

### Pharmacy Information /Medications    La farmacia/los medicamentos
I need …., Necesito…
the name of your pharmacy, el nombre de su farmacia.
the address/telephone number of your pharmacy, la dirección/ el número de teléfono de su farmacia
I need a list of…, Yo necesito una lista de…
your medications/vitamins, sus medicatmentos/vitaminas

### Medical insurance Information, Información sobre el seguro medico
Can I please see your…, ¿Me permite ver su…
I need a photocopy of your…, Necesito un fotocopia de su …
Medical ID card, tarjeta de seguro médico
Medicaid / medicare card, tarjeta de Medicaid/medicare
Who is paying the bill…?, ¿Quién paga la cuenta…?
the patient or the insurance?, el paciente o el seguro?
What is your …?, ¿Cuál es su…?
primary /secondary insurance, seguro principal / seguro secundario
policy /policy number, póliza (nombre de la póliza) / número de póliza
Do you have…?, ¿Tiene…..?
a deductible/a copayment/co-insurance, deducible/copago/coseguro
What is …, ¿Cuál es …?
the name of the insured, el nombre del asegurado
the address of the insured, la dirección del asegurado

### General Instructions to the Patient, Instrucciones al paciente
Please enter. Pase, por favor.
Please take a seat. Tome un asiento, por favor.
I will be with you shortly. Le atiendo en seguida.
Fill out the form, please. Llene la planilla, por favor
Sign and date the … please. Firme y feche …, por favor.
form, la   planilla
authorization form, la autorización
consent form, el consentimiento
**HIPAA consent form**, la autorización para divulgar informacón médica de conformidad con HIPAA

### Height & Weight Information
Height, estatura
Weight, peso
How tall are you?, ¿Cuánto mide?
How much do you weigh?, ¿Cuánto pesa?

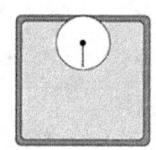

### Place of employment/school, Lugar de trabajo
Name of your employer name of your school, Nombre de su empleador/ escuela
What is your employer's/school's…?, ¿Cuál es …de su empleador/escuela?
address, la dirección
telephone number, el número de teléfono
e-mail, dirección de correo electrónico
What is your occupation?, ¿Cúal es su ocupación?

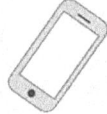

### Emergency Contact, Contacto en caso de emergencia
I need …of your emergency contact. Yo necesito…de su contacto de emergencia.
the name/ address/ telephone number, el nombre/la dirección/ el número de teléfono

### Doctor Information
Who is your primary doctor?, ¿Quién es su médico de cabecera/ médico primario?
What is your primary doctor's…?, ¿Cuál es …de su médico de cabecera?
Address/ telephone number/ e-mail, la dirección/el número de teléfono/la dirección de correo electrónico

### Doctor's Appointments, Pedir citas con el médico
You need.., Necesita ..
an appointment with the doctor, pedir una cita/hacer una cita con el médico
to change your appointment, cambiar su hora de la cita
to confirm your appointment, confirmar su cita
Your doctor's appointment is at ____ am/pm, Su cita médica es a la/ las _____ de la mañana/tarde/noche
Your doctor's appointment is…, Su cita está …
confirmed /cancelled/rescheduled, confirmada / cancelada/cambiada

# PRESENT MEDICAL HISTORY (ILLNESSES)  HISTORIA MEDICA- ENFERMEDADES

Present medical history (illnesses), Historia médica enfermedades

Do you drink alcohol? ¿Usted bebe alcohol?
Do you use recreational drugs? ¿Ingiere drogas recreativas?
Do you smoke? ¿Usted fuma?
What are your hobbies? ¿Cuáles son sus pasatiempos?

Are you pregnant? ¿Está embarazada?
Have you ever been pregnant?, ¿Ha estado embarazada?
Are you sexually active? ¿Está activo(a) sexualmente?
How many sexual partners do you have? ¿Cuántas parejas sexuales tiene?
Do you have a sexually transmitted infection? ¿Tiene alguna infección de transmisión sexual?

Do you have allergies...? ¿Tiene alergias...?
to any food/any medicine/any antibiotic? a algún alimento/a alguna medicina/algún antibiótico?

Have you ever had any of the following illnesses? ¿Ha tenido alguna de las siguientes enfermedades?

Has any member of your family had any of the following illnesses?¿Algún miembro de su familia ha tenido alguna de estas enfermedades?

Is there anyone in your family with ... ? ¿Hay alguien en su familia con ... ?

·Alzheimer's disease, La enfermedad Alzheimer
·blood clots, coágulos de sangre
·cancer, cáncer
·type of cancer, tipo de cáncer
·diabetes mellitus/diabetes type 1/diabetes type 2, diabetes mellitus/ la diabetes tipo 1/la diabetes tipo 2
·epileptic attacks, ataques epilépticos
·heart attack, ataque de corazón
·heart disease, enfermedad cardiovascular
·heart problems, problemas del corazón
·high blood pressure, presión sanguinea alta/la presión arterial alta

- high cholesterol, colesterol alto
- migraines, migrañas
- Multiple Sclerosis, Esclerosis Múltiple
- paralysis, parálisis cerebral
- stroke, derrame cerebral or infarto

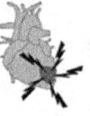  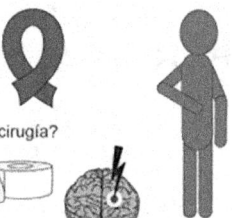

Have you had any surgery? ¿Ha tenido alguna operación/ cirugía?
Other hospitalizations? ¿Alguna hospitalización?
Other serious illnesses? ¿Alguna enfermedad grave?
Other serious injuries? ¿Alguna herida grave?

Vaccine Information, Información sobre sus vacunas

Do you have all your vaccinations completed?/Do you have all your vaccines? ¿*Tiene sus vacunas completas? ¿Tiene todas sus vacunas?*

Have you received the vaccine for... ¿Recibió la vacuna contra...?
...Hepatitis A ? Hepatitis B? ...la hepatitis A? ...la hepatitis B?
...pneumococcal?...la neumocócica?
...chickenpox? ...la varicela?
...MMR? (Measles, Mumps, Rubella), contra MMR? ...triple vírica? (el sarampión, las paperas y la rubéola)
...shingles? ...la culebrilla?
...smallpox? ...la viruela?
...rabies? ...la rabia?
...COVID 19? ....Covid 19?

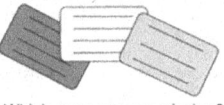 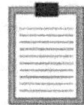

Which one are you missing? Which ones are you missing? ¿Cuál le falta? ¿Cuales le falta?

Do you have your vaccinations records (card)? ¿Tiene su registro (cartilla) de vacunación?

## OJO take note: DIALECT EXPRESSIONS

Stuffy nose: La nariz tupida (El Caribe), La nariz tapada (Mexico)
The form: La planilla, el formulario (El Caribe), la forma (Mexico)
The belly: La barriga, la pipa (El Caribe), la panza (Mexico)
Right now: Ahora vs ahorita, which is just the opposite in El Caribe, Mexico and Central America)

**Contributed by Joanna Rios, PhD**

## DOCTOR'S VISIT — PATIENT INFORMATION — PATIENT HISTORY

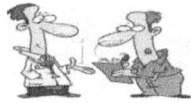

Physical exam-questions to the patient, Examen físico-preguntas al paciente

What brings you here? ¿Qué le trae por aquí?
How can I help you? ¿En que puedo servirle?
What's wrong? ¿Qué le pasa?
How are you? ¿Cómo está Usted?
How do you feel? ¿Cómo se siente?
Do you feel well? Do you feel sick? ¿Se siente bien? ¿Se siente enfermo/a?
Do you have any discomforts? ¿Tiene Usted malestar/ molestias?
Everything is normal. OR All is well. Todo es normal OR Todo está bien.
Are you allergic to anything? ¿Es usted alérgico a algo?
Can you raise your arms? ¿Puede levantar los brazos?
Do you have problems chewing /swallowing? ¿Tiene problemas para masticar?/para tragar

OJO 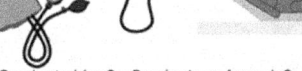: In 1980, 18-year-old Willie Ramirez was admitted to a Florida hospital in a comatose state. He had gone to a fast food restaurant and got very sick afterwards. Ramirez's family believed he was suffering from food poisoning. His friends and family explained to the admitting doctors in Spanish that Willie was 'intoxicado'. A bilingual staff member translated 'intoxicado' as 'intoxicated.' (In Cuban Spanish, 'intoxicado' is used to describe a person who has ingested bad food or drink. In English 'intoxicated' refers to drug or alcohol abuse). The doctors erroneously treated Willie for a drug overdose. They failed to diagnose his actual condition, which was an intracerebral hemorrhage. The delay in diagnosis and treatment resulted in Willie Ramirez becoming a quadriplegic. This medical translation error resulted in a $71 million lawsuit. In her book, "An Intoxicating Error: Mistranslation, Medical Malpractice, and Prejudice," Gail Price-Wise discusses the factors other than the translation error (prejudice, stereotyping and cultural nuances) that contributed to this malpractice case.

Instructions to patients, Instrucciones a los pacientes

Put on this gown. Póngase esta bata.
Undress from the waist up/waist down. Desvístase de la cintura para arriba/ para abajo.
Take off your clothes completely. Quítese toda la ropa.
Sit on the table. Siéntese sobre la mesa.
Relax, please. Relájese, por favor.
Turn face down/face up. Póngase boca abajo / boca arriba.
Open your mouth. Abra la boca.
Cough, please. Tosa, por favor.
Swallow, please. Trague, por favor.
Come with a full bladder. Venga con la vejiga llena.
Come with an empty stomach. Venga en ayunas.
Collect and bring your urine. Acumule y traiga la orina.
Breathe in/Breathe out. Respire or Inhale/Exhale, por favor.
Breathe quickly/Breathe slowly. Respire rápido/Respire lento/despacio.
Take a deep breath/Breathe deeply. Respire hondo y profundamente/Respire profundo.
Hold your breath. Aguante la respiración.
Stick your tongue out. Saque la lengua.
Keep your eyes to the front. Mire hacia el frente.
Extend your arms. Extienda los brazos.
Bend your knees. Doble las rodillas.
Tell me when you feel the pain. Dígame cuando sienta dolor.
Point to where you feel the pain. Señale donde le duele.
Lie down on the table. Acuéstese sobre la mesa.
Lie on your side. Acuéstese de medio lado.

# VITAL SIGNS 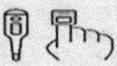 LOS SIGNOS VITALES

Vital signs, Signos vitales

| Body temperature (abbreviation: TC), La temperatura corporal |
|---|
| hyperthermia, hipertermia<br>hypothermia, hipotermia |
| Temperature measurement locations, Lugares de medición de la temperatura<br>Orally, Por vía oral.<br>Rectal, En el recto (vía rectal).<br>Axillary, En la axila.<br>By ear, En el oído.<br>Skin, En la piel. |
| Types of the thermometers:<br>Tipos de termómetros: |

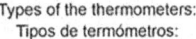

Digital thermometer, termómetro digital
Glass thermometer, termómetro de vidrio
Ear thermometer, termómetro de oído
Infrared thermometer, termómetro infrarrojo
Non contact thermometer, termómetro sin contacto

| Pulse (heart rate) (abbreviation: FC), Pulso arterial y frecuencia cardiaca |
|---|
| bradycardia, bradicardia<br>tachycardia, taquicardia |
| The pulse, El pulso<br>places to take the pulse, lugares para tomar el pulso |

 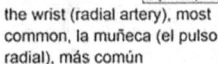

the wrist (radial artery), most common, la muñeca (el pulso radial), más común

-temporal superficial artery, arteria temporal superficial
-carotid aertery, arteria carótida
-subclavian artery, arteria subclavia
-brachial artery arteria braquial
-axial artery, arteria axilar
-femoral artery, arteria femoral
-popliteal artery, arteria poplitea
-posterior tibial artery, arteria tibial posterior
-dorsal artery of the foot, arteria pedia

| Respiration rate, Frecuencia respiratoria |
|---|
| -dyspnea, disnea<br>-eupnea, eupnea<br>-bradypnea, bradipnea<br>-tachypnea, taquipnea<br>-apnea, apnea<br>-ortopnea, ortopnea<br>-hyperpnea, hiperpnea<br>-hyperventilation, hiperventilación<br>-hypoventilation, hipoventilación |

| Blood pressure (abbreviation: TA), Tensión arterial |
|---|
| hypertension/hypotension, hipertensión/hipotensión |

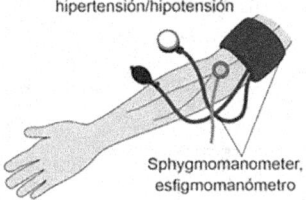

Sphygmomanometer, esfigmomanómetro

| Oxygen saturation, saturación de oxígeno en sangre |
|---|

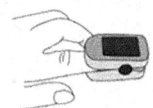

Oximeter, el oxímetro

| range, rango | values, valores |
|---|---|
| normal, normal | 95-100% |
| mild hypoxia, hipoxia leve | 91-94% |
| moderate hypoxia, hipoxia moderada | 86-90% |
| severe hypoxia, hipoxia grave | 86% or less, menos |

| VITAL SIGN<br>SIGNO VITAL | REQUESTING PERMISSION<br>PEDIRLE PERMISO AL PACIENTE | GIVING RESULTS TO THE PATIENT<br>DARLE RESULTADOS AL PACIENTE |
|---|---|---|
| The pulse-el pulso | Can I take your pulse? ¿Me permite tomar su pulso? ¿Puedo tomarle el pulso? | Your pulse is ___ beats per minute. Su latido está en ___ latidos por minuto. You have a fast/slow/normal/irregular/pulse. Su pulso es rápido/lento/normal/irregular. Your pulse is __ per minute. Su pulso está en __ por minuto. |
| Heart beat-latidos cardíacos | Can I check your heart rate? ¿Me permite comprobar su ritmo cardíaco? | Your heart beat is irregular/fast/slow. Sus latidos cardíacos son irregulares/rápidos/lentos. |
| The oxygen-el oxígeno | Can I measure your oxygen level? ¿Me permite medirle el oxígeno? | Your oxygen is 98%. Su oxígeno está en 98% (por ciento). An oxygen concentration of __ is normal. Una concentración de oxígeno en ___ es normal. |
| Blood pressure-la presión arterial | Can I please take your blood pressure? ¿Me permite tomar su presión arterial? | Your pressure is 120/80. Su presión está en 120 sobre ochenta. You have high / low/ normal blood pressure. Usted tiene presión arterial alta/ baja/ normal. |
| Temperature-temperatura | Can I take your temperature? ¿Me permite tomarle la temperatura? | Your temperature is ___ degrees. Su temperatura está en ___ grados. You have a low grade fever. Tiene febrícula. You have a moderate/high/continuous/intermittent fever. Tiene una fiebre moderada/alta/continua/intermitente. |

# MEDICATIONS / MEDICAMENTOS

Medications: a list of your prescriptions,
Medicamentos: una lista de sus recetas

 analgesics, los analgésicos

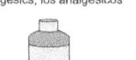 antacids, los antiácidos

 antibiotics, los antibióticos

 antidepressant, el antidepresivo

 antihistamines, los antihistamínicos

 antiseptics, los antisépticos

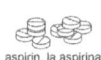 aspirin, la aspirina

 cortisone, la cortisona

cough syrup, el jarabe para la tos

cream, la pomada

decongestant, el descongestionante

cold relief medicine, el antigripal

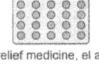 diuretic, el diurético

 drops (for the eyes), las gotas (para los ojos)

 estrogen, el estrógeno

expectorant, el expectorante

 inhaler, el inhalador

insulin, la insulina

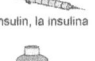 laxative, el laxante

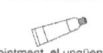 ointment, el ungüento

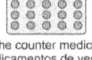 over the counter medications, los medicamentos de venta libre

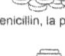 penicillin, la penicilina

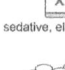 sedative, el sedante

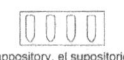 steroid, el esteroide

 suppository, el supositorio

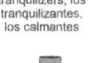 tranquilizers, los tranquilizantes, los calmantes

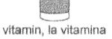 vitamin, la vitamina

Units of measure, Unidades de medida

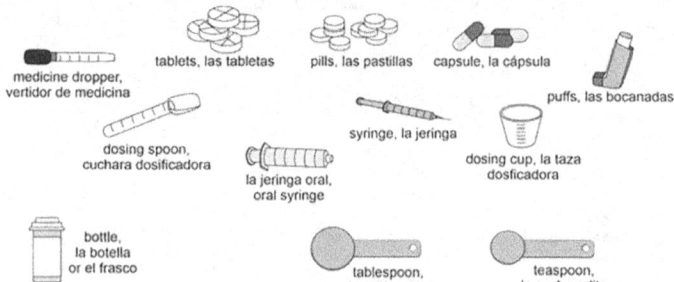

Medicine storage, Almacenamiento de medicamentos

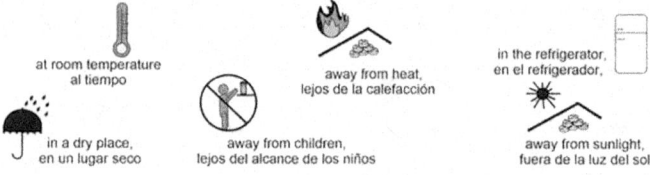

# INSTRUCTIONS FOR TAKING MEDICATIONS
# INSTRUCCIONES PARA MEDICAMENTOS

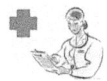

Instructions for medication, Instrucciones para medicamentos

Prescription Label, La etiqueta

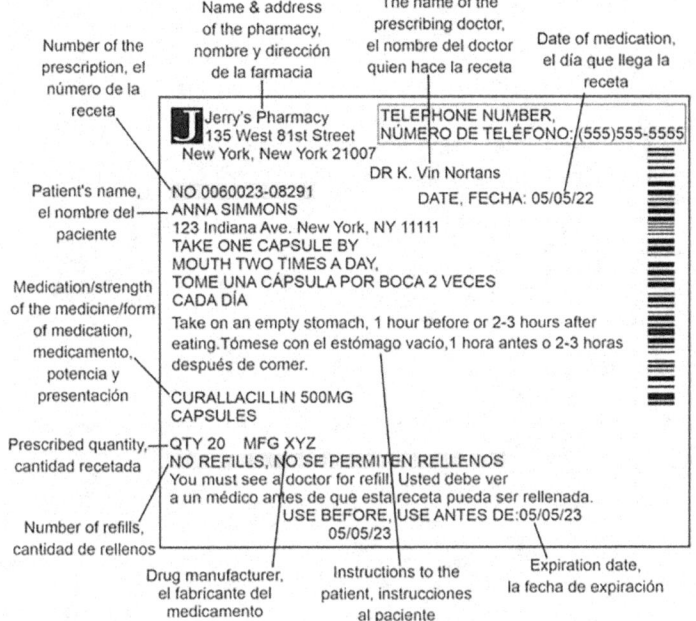

Instructions for medication, Instrucciones para medicamentos

Pharmacy/Rx vocabulary, La farmacia/ las recetas vocabulario
generic version, la versión genérica
medications, los medicamentos
on-line pharmacy, farmacia por correo
over-the-counter medications, la recetas de venta libre
pharmacist, el/la farmaceútico,a
pharmacy, la farmacia
prescription, receta
prescription drugs, los medicamentos con receta

Method of ingestion, Como ingerir
To swallow, tragar
To chew, masticar
To put drops in eyes, poner gotas
To inhale, inhalar
Inhaler, el inhalador
Injectable, el inyectable
Nasal use, uso nasal
Nasal inhalers, inhaladores nasales
Oral inhalers, inhaladores orales
Oral use, uso oral
Pump, bomba/bombilla

calendario, calendar

Frequency, Frecuencia
Take this medicine…, Tome esta medicina
____times a day, ____veces al día
Every day…every other day….., cada día ….un día sí, un día no, cada tercer día
Every___hours, cada ___ horas
in the morning/evening, por la mañana/por la noche.
Before eating /with each meal/after eating…, antes de comer/con cada comida/ después de comer

Warnings, Advertencias
Avoid staying in the sun while taking this medicine. Evite exponerse al sol mientras esté tomando la medicina
Chew pills before swallowing. Masticar antes de tragar.
Keep in a cool place. Consérvese en un lugar fresco y seco
Keep out of reach of children. Manténga los medicamentos fuera del alcance de los niños
Keep refrigerated. Manténgase refrigerado/a.
Shake well before using. Agítese bien antes de usarlo.
You need to take all of the medicine. Necesita tomar toda la medicina.

Side effects, Efectos secundarios
This medicine can cause..., Este medicamento puede causar
diarrhea, diarrhea
dizziness, mareos
drowsiness, somnolencia
dry mouth, boca seca
stomach pain, dolor estomacal
This medicine can impair driving, Este medicamento puede afectar la capacidad para conducir

Refills/Expiration, Rellenos/Fecha de caducidad
Expired medication, medicamentos caducos
Expiration date, Fecha de caducidad/fecha de vencimiento
This medicine does not have refills. Esta receta no puede rellenarse.
Throw out after _____, Deséchese después de.........
There can be _____ refills. Esta receta puede _____ rellenados
Don't use after _____, No use después de_____

---

OJO take note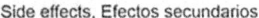: A study evaluated the accuracy of computer-generated translation of medicine labels in Spanish. **(Accuracy of Computer-Generated, Spanish-Language Medicine Labels** by Iman Sharif, MD, MPH;Julia Tse, BA, Pediatrics (2010) 125 (5): 960–965.) The research was conducted in pharmacies around Bronx, New York and involved 316 independent pharmacies. Researchers evaluated 76 medicine labels generated by 13 different computer programs commonly used by pharmacies. The study found an overall error rate of 50 percent.
- One example of a prescription mistranslation was that of a man with a heart condition whose prescription stated that his medication should be taken **once a day**. The English term **once** is read as "once" (on-se), which is the Spanish word for the number 11. As the English instruction was retained in the medicine label, the **patient mistakenly took 11 pills** rather than just one pill per day.
- Misspelling in the translations created hazardous and potentially life-threatening errors. For example, the word "poca", which means "little", instead of the word " boca", which means "mouth". Another example of a misspelled error is "dos besos", which means "two kisses", instead of "dos veces", which means "two times".
- Poor translations specifically cited in the study included: "Take 1.2 aldia give dropperfuls with juice eleven to day." "Taking 0.6 mL 2 times to the day by the little with juice." "Apply to affected area twice to the indicated day like."

# X-RAYS & TESTS - RADIOGRAFIAS / ANALISIS

X-ray & tests, Radiografias/analisis

biopsy, una biopsia
blood culture, un cultivo de sangre
blood test, un análisis de sangre
CAT scan, una tomografía axial computarizada
colonoscopy, una colonoscopía
EEG, un electroencefalograma
(EKG) electrocardiogram, un electrocardiograma
endoscopy, una endoscopía
MRI, una imagen de resonancia magnética
mammogram, una mamografía
Pap smear, un Papanicolau

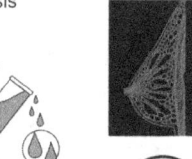
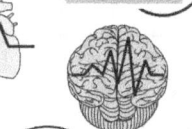
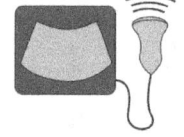 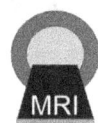

laproscopy, una laproscopía
stress test, un examen de estrés
sputum test, un análisis de sputum
ultrasound, un ultrasonido
urine test, un análisis de orina

X-rays of the…, radiografias de…
head..chest..leg..hand..knee, la cabeza..el pecho..la pierna..la rodilla

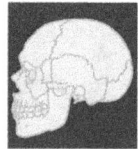 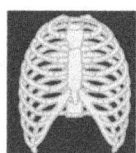 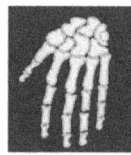 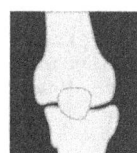

| The hospital- Facilities and Departments | 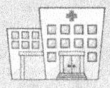 | El hospital –lugares y departamentos |
|---|---|---|

Hospital departments, Departamentos del hospital

The Ward, La sala de

Anesthesiology, anestesiología

Cardiology, cardiología

Dermatology, dermatología

Emergency, urgencias

Gastroenterology, gastroenterología

Hematology, hematología

Intensive Care Unit, ICU-(la) Unidad de Cuidados Intensivos (UCI)/(la)
Unidad de Vigilancia Intensiva (UVI)

Internal medicine, medicina interna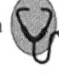

Nephrology, nefrología,

Neonatal, neonatología

Obstetrics & gynecology, obstetricia y ginecología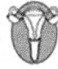

Oncology, oncología

Ophthalmology, oftalmología

Otolaryngology, otorrinolaringología

Pediatrics, pediatría

Pulmonary, neumologia

Traumatology, traumatología

Hospital support areas, áreas de apoyo hospitalario
Administrative offices, áreas administrativas
Admissions, La admisión
Doctor's office, consultorio del médico
Human Resources, recursos humanos
Laboratory, el laboratorio
The pharmacy, la farmacia
Radiology, la radiología
Recovery, la sala de recuperación
Reception area, la recepción
Waiting room, la sala de espera

Hospital parts, Las partes del hospital
Directory, el directorio
Entrance, La entrada
Exit, la salida
Parking, el estacionamiento
Patient's room, el cuarto del paciente
El piso número____, floor number _____

## Medical personnel, Personales médicos

lab technician, el/la técnico/a de laboratorio
anesthesiologist, el/la anestesiólogo/a
dentist, el/la dentista
doctor, el doctor/la doctora/el médico/la médica
ENT doctor, el/la especialista de garganta, naríz y oídos (otorrinolaringólogo)
family doctor, el/la médico de familia
gynecologist, el/la ginecólogo/a
midwife, (la) matrona
neurologist, el/la neurólogo/a
nurse, el/la enfermero/a
obstetrician, el/la obstetra
ophthalmologist, el/la oculista, (el/la) oftalmólogo/a
oncologist, el/la oncólogo/a
pediatrician, el/la pediatra
psychologist, el/la psicólogo/a
psychiatrist, el/la psiquiatro/a
surgeon, el/la cirujano/cirujana
x-ray technician, el/la técnico(a) de rayos x

## Emergency Professions & Providers, Profesiones de emergencia

emergency care provider, el proveedor de servicios de emergencia
fire captain, el capitán de bomberos
fire chief, el jefe de bomberos
fire department, el departamento de bomberos
fire station, la estación de bomberos
fire fighter, el/la bombero/a
first responder, el/la que responde primero a emergencias
health care provider, el/la proveedor/a de cuidado médico
paramedic, el/la paramédico/a
police department, el departamento de policía
rescue worker, el/la trabajador/a de rescate
EMT/first responder, el/la técnico/a de emergencias,

## Medical equipment, Equipo médico

ambulance, la ambulancia
bandage, el vendaje
bed, la cama
bed pan, el orinal, la chata
cast, el yeso
crutches, las muletas
drip, el suero
gloves, los guantes
needle, la aguja
mask, la mascarilla
painkiller, el analgésico
stretcher, la camilla
scalpel, el bisturí
stethoscope, el estetoscopio
syringe, la jeringa
vaccine, la vacuna

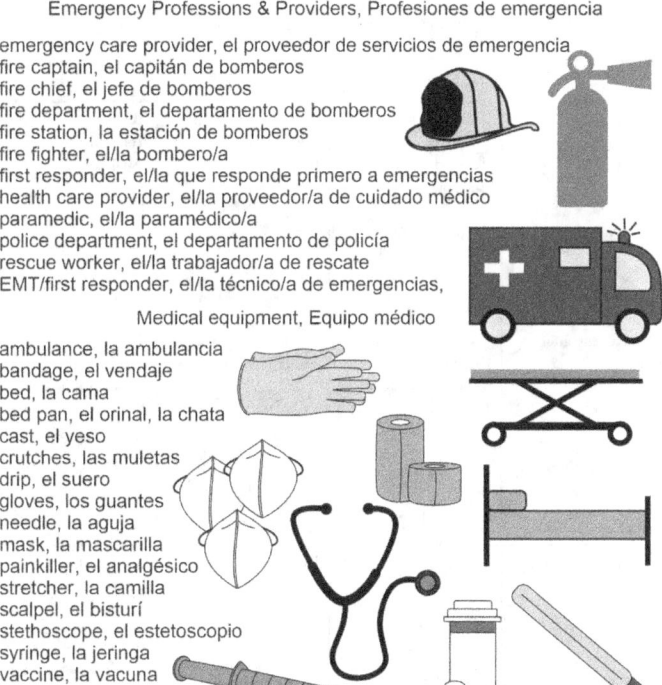

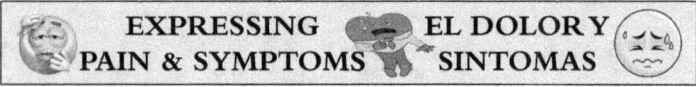

# EXPRESSING PAIN & SYMPTOMS — EL DOLOR Y SINTOMAS

## THE NOUN- EL DOLOR –THE PAIN

The noun 'dolor' means 'pain'. One way to express pain is to use the verb *'tener'*. Use the construction **tener dolor de + body part**. This literally means: To have pain of + body part. Example: Tengo dolor de la oreja. My ear hurts. Literally: I have pain of the ear.

**OJO** take note. The verb tener-to have- is an irregular verb. The following are the conjugations: yo tengo, tú tienes, él, ella, Usted tiene, nosotros tenemos, vosotros tenéis, ellos, Ustedes tienen.

| To have a headache. Tener dolor de cabeza. | To have a sore throat. Tener dolor de la garganta. | To have chest pain. Tener dolor del pecho. | To have a backache. Tener dolor de espalda |
|---|---|---|---|
| To have a stomach ache. Tener dolor de estómago. | To have a pain in the hand(s). Tener dolor de la mano. | To have foot pain. Tener dolor de pies. | To have shoulder pain. Tener dolor del hombro. |
| To have knee pain. Tener dolor de la rodilla. | To have a toothache. Tener dolor de las muelas. | To have a neck ache. Tener dolor del cuello. | To have leg pain. Tener dolor de la pierna. |

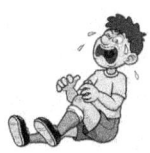 **THE VERB DOLER-TO HURT**

The verb *doler* is an o: ue stem changing verb. The two most commonly used forms are the third person singular *duele* or the third person plural *duelen*. The *doler* construction is similar to the *gustar* construction. It does not follow the English construction where the subject is the person experiencing the pain. In Spanish, the subject of the sentence is the part or parts of the body that hurt.

For example : In English we say: My hands hurt. In Spanish we say: Me duelen las manos. Literally: The hands hurt me.

## 3- PART CONSTRUCTION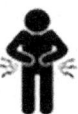

**Indirect object pronoun (IDOP) + duele or duelen + body part (IDOP=recipient of pain)**

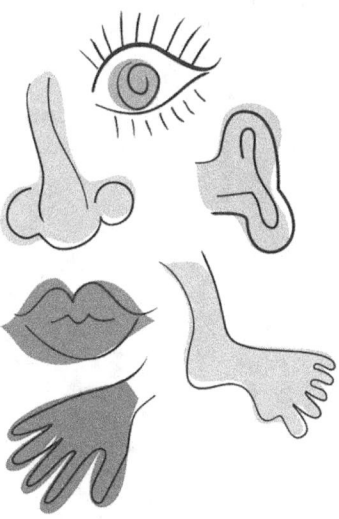

## IF ONE BODY PART HURTS:

| IDOP (who is feeling the pain) **me, te, le, nos, os, les** | + duele | + body part | |
|---|---|---|---|

## IF MORE THAN ONE BODY PART HURTS:

| IDOP (who is feeling the pain) **me, te, le, nos, os, les** | + duelen | + body part | |
|---|---|---|---|

OJO take note The third person IDOP, *le* can mean 'to him', 'to her', 'to you (formal)', to it (such as a pet). To determine which person it is referring to, use context (what came before) or a clarifier. Example- Le duele la cabeza *a Juan*. Juan's head hurts. The third person plural IDOP, *les*, can mean 'to them' or 'to you (all)'. Meaning is determined by context (what came before) or a clarifier. Example: Les duele la cabeza *a Juan y Julia*. Their (Juan's & Julia's head hurts.

**OJO** *take note* You do not use a possessive to refer to the body part. You use the definite article (el, la, los, las). The recipient of pain is expressed in the IDOP (Indirect Object Pronoun).

Examples:

*My hand hurts.* Me duele la mano. *Literal translation:* The hand hurts me.

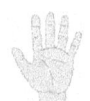

*My hands hurt.* Me duelen las manos. Literal translation: The hands hurt me.

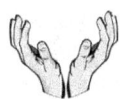

Your (familiar) nose hurts. Te duele la naríz. Literal translation: The nose hurts you (familiar)

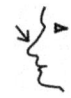

His/her/your (formal) foot hurts. Le duele la pierna. *Literal translation:* The foot hurts him/her or you formal.

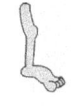

His/her/your (formal) feet hurt. Le duelen las piernas. *Literal translation:* The feet hurt him / her or you formal.

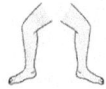

Our ear hurts. Nos duele el oído. *Literal translation:* The ear hurts us.

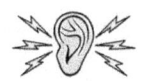

Our ears hurt. Nos duelen los oídos. *Literal translation:* The ears hurt us.

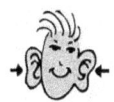

Their or your (plural) toe hurts. Les duele el dedo de pie. *Literal translation:* The toe hurts them or you(all).

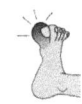

Their or your (all of you) toes hurt. Les duelen los dedos de pie. *Literal translation:* The toes hurt them or you (all).

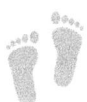

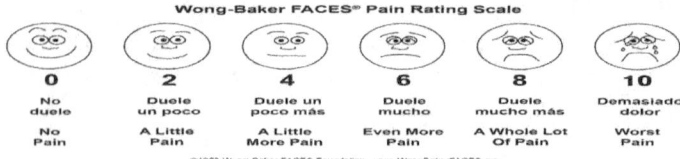

**OJO** take note The Wong–Baker Faces Pain Rating Scale was developed by Donna Wong and Connie Baker in 1983. It is a tool for self- assessment of pain using faces (0 or no pain to 10 worst pain). This was originally developed for children. However, it is useful for patients with language barriers and has been translated in various languages. (Wikipedia)

# PAIN ASSESSMENT & TYPES OF PAIN 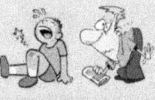 LA EVALUACION DEL DOLOR Y TIPOS DE DOLOR

Patient's Pain Assessment, Evaluación del dolor del paciente

Patient's History of Pain, La historia del dolor del paciente
How long has it hurt you? ¿Cúanto tiempo hace que le duele?
When did the pain start? ¿Cuándo empezó el dolor?
Since when have you had the pain? ¿Desde cuando tiene el dolor?

Patient's Pain Location, El lugar del dolor del paciente
Where does it hurt? ¿Dónde le duele?
Point to where it hurts, please. Señale donde le duele, por favor.
Does it hurt anywhere else? ¿Le duele en otro lugar?
Does the pain move anywhere? ¿Se traslada el dolor a otro lugar?
Does it hurt when I press here? ¿Le duele cuando le aprieto aquí?
Where does it hurt most? ¿Dónde le duele más?

Patient's Pain Frequency & Duration, Frecuencia y duración del dolor del paciente

Is the pain... ¿Es el dolor...?
Constant, constante
Comes and goes, va y viene
Every day?, todos los días
How long does the pain last? ¿Cuánto tiempo dura el dolor?

Patient's Type of Pain, El tipo del dolor del paciente
Is the pain .... ¿El dolor es ...
light, leve
moderate, moderado
intense, ntenso
severe, severo
unbearable, insoportable

How much does it hurt you? ¿Cuánto le duele?
How much does it hurt on a scale of 1-10? ¿Cuánto le duele en una escala de uno a diez?
How long does the pain hurt? ¿Cuándo le dura el dolor?

Factors that aggravate or relieve the pain, Los factores que empeoran/ mejoran el dolor
What makes the pain start? ¿Qué hace que su dolor comience?
What makes it hurt less? ¿Qué alivia el dolor?
What makes it hurt more? ¿Qué hace empeorar el dolor?
Is the pain worse when you... ¿Es el dolor peor cuando ... ?
    feel stressed? está estresado
    you work? está trabajando
    you sit down? se siente/está sentado
    you get up? se levanta

As Impact of pain on patient, El impacto del dolor al paciente
Does the pain affect....? ¿El dolor afecta ...?
your appetite, ... su apetito?
your work, ... su trabajo?
your social life, ...su vida social?
Has the pain ever affected your sleep? ¿El dolor lo ha despertado de dormir?

# AILMENTS—SYMPTOMS 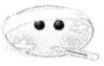 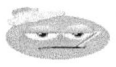 DOLENCIAS Y SINTOMAS

| | | | | |
|---|---|---|---|---|
| broken leg- *pierna rota* | bump-*roncha* | blood clot- *coágulo de sangre* | bruise-*moretón* | bite-*mordedura* |
| cough-*tos* | constipated- *estreñido* | cut-*cortadura* | chills- *escalofríos* | chicken pox- *varicela* |
| cold-*catarro, resfriado* | cramp-*calambre* | dizzy-*mareado*  dizzy spells-*mareos* | diarrhea-*diarrea* | dry mouth-*la boca seca* |
| fever-*fiebre* | flu-*gripe* | fatigue or weakness  *fatiga or tener debilidad* | fracture-*fractura* | heartburn- *acidez estomacal or ardor* |
| high/low blood pressure- *presión arterial alta/baja* | hay fever-*fiebre del heno or* allergies-*alergías* | hiccups-<u>*tener hipo*</u> | Hemorrhoids- *hemorroides* | insect bite  *picadura de insecto* |
| itch  *picazón/ comezón/picor* | insomnia- *insomnio* | kidney stones- *cálculos renales* | lump-*bulto* | to bleed-*sangrar* to cough up blood-*toser sangre* |

| laryngitis- *laringitis* | mouth sores- *úlceras bucales* | measles- *sarampión* | mumps-*paperas* | nausea-*náusea* |
|---|---|---|---|---|
| numbness- *adormecimiento* | nose bleed- *hemorragia nasal* | palpitations- *palpitaciones* | rash-*sarpullido* | staggering- *tambaleo* |
| swelling- *hinchazón* | shortness of breath *falta de aire* | sun stroke- *insolación* | sunburn- *quemadura de sol* | seizures-*ataques epilépticos* |
| tingling- *cosquilleo* | ulcer-*úlcera* | wart-*verruga* | vomiting- *vómitos* | shingles-*herpes zoster, culebrilla* |

OJO *take note* **FOLK ILLNESS,** otherwise referred to as a culture-bound syndrome, or a culture-specific syndrome, is a disease recognizable only by a specific culture or society. Some examples of folk illness or culture-bound syndrome / culture-specific syndroms in Latin America are: ***empacho, susto or mal de susto, nervios, caída de mollera and mal de ojo. Empacho*** is a Central American folk illness, referring to gastrointestinal issues. It is characterized by obstruction of the stomach and or intestine. The symptoms of **empacho** include abdominal pain, bloating, nausea, vomiting, lethargy and diarrhea. ***Empacho*** is believed to be caused by food sticking to the intestinal wall due to eating certain foods at incorrect times, swallowing gum, swallowing too much saliva, among other things. Another folk illness common to Latin American cultures is **susto. *Susto* or *mal de susto*** can be medically diagnosed as reactive depression or a post-traumatic stress syndrome caused by a traumatic event. Symptoms of **susto** are nervousness, fever, depression, diarrhea and lethargy. Another folk illness similar to **susto** is **nervios. Nervios** can consist of trembling, shouting, seizures, fainting spells. ***Caída de mollera*** refers to "fallen fontanel" and many times is attributed to maternal neglect. The medical diagnosis of ***caída de mollera*** is dehydration. This is caused by pulling the baby from the breast or bottle too quickly or holding the baby incorrectly or letting the baby fall. A very common Latin American folk-illness is **mal de ojo.** The translation of **mal de ojo** is an 'evil eye'. [From Spanish mal illness + de of + ojo an eye] (Oxford Reference) **Mal de ojo** is common to many Mediterranean countries and Latino communities. **Mal de ojo** is caused by the jealousy or envy of admirers. The symptoms can range from irritability, crying, fever. Common symptoms of **mal de ojo** are insomnia, diarrhea, vomiting and fever.

| FIRST AID  | PRIMEROS AUXILIOS |
| --- | --- |
| FIRST AID KIT  | BOTIQUIN DE PRIMEROS AUXILIOS |

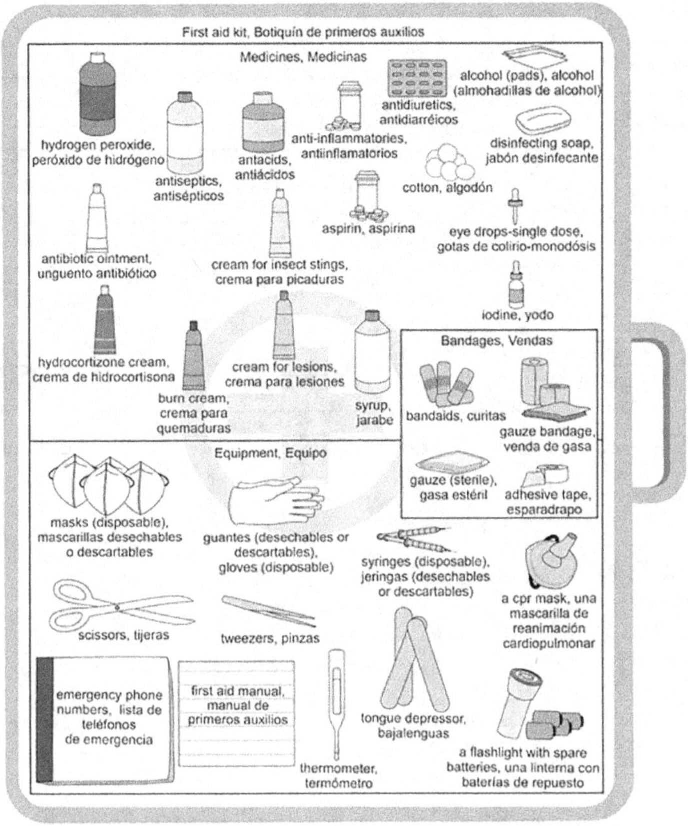

First aid kit, Botiquín de primeros auxilios

**Medicines, Medicinas**

- hydrogen peroxide, peróxido de hidrógeno
- antiseptics, antisépticos
- antacids, antiácidos
- anti-inflammatories, antiinflamatorios
- aspirin, aspirina
- antidiuretics, antidiarréicos
- alcohol (pads), alcohol (almohadillas de alcohol)
- disinfecting soap, jabón desinfectante
- cotton, algodón
- eye drops-single dose, gotas de colirio-monodósis
- antibiotic ointment, unguento antibiótico
- cream for insect stings, crema para picaduras
- iodine, yodo
- hydrocortizone cream, crema de hidrocortisona
- burn cream, crema para quemaduras
- cream for lesions, crema para lesiones
- syrup, jarabe

**Bandages, Vendas**

- bandaids, curitas
- gauze bandage, venda de gasa
- gauze (sterile), gasa estéril
- adhesive tape, esparadrapo

**Equipment, Equipo**

- masks (disposable), mascarillas desechables o descartables
- guantes (desechables or descartables), gloves (disposable)
- syringes (disposable), jeringas (desechables or descartables)
- a cpr mask, una mascarilla de reanimación cardiopulmonar
- scissors, tijeras
- tweezers, pinzas
- emergency phone numbers, lista de teléfonos de emergencia
- first aid manual, manual de primeros auxilios
- tongue depressor, bajalenguas
- thermometer, termómetro
- a flashlight with spare batteries, una linterna con baterías de repuesto

# First Aid Vocabulary  Vocabulario para primeros auxilios

First aid, Primeros auxilios

| | |
|---|---|
| allergic reaction, reacción alérgica | |
| bites (animal), mordeduras de animales | |
| burns, quemaduras | |
| chocking, atragamiento | |
| coughing or throwing up blood Tos con sangre o vómitos de sangre | |
| drowing, ahogamiento | |
| electrocution, electrocución | |
| fractures/broken bones, fracturas (huesos quebrados) fracturas de huesos | |
| frost-bite, congelación | |
| gunshot wound, herida de bala | |
| hemorrhages (nasal /internal/external), hemorragias (hemorragia nasal/ interna/externa) | |
| intoxication (alcohol/medications/gas/carbon monoxide), intoxicación por alcohol/medicamentos/gases | |
| loss of vital signs, pérdida de signos vitales | |
| low blood sugar, hipoglucemia | |
| overdose of drug or alcohol, sobredosis de drogas o alcohol | |
| poisoning, envenenamiento | |
| seizure/epileptic attack, convulsión/ataque epiléptico | |
| stings/insect/jellyfish, picaduras (insectos/medusas) | |
| stab wound, puñalada | |
| twists or spains, torceduras o esquinces | |

# FIRST AID 911 -  Primeros Auxilios-emergencia 911

## Conducta PAS, First aid code of conduct

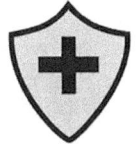 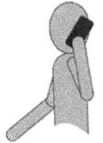 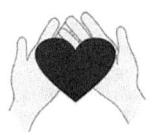

**proteger,** protect the emergency zone    **avisar,** advise 911    **socorrer,** help the victim

First aid procedures, Procedimientos de primeros auxilios

| | |
|---|---|
| abdominal thrusts, compresiones abdominales | |
| basic life support, soporte vital básico | |
| cardiopulmonary rescusitation, reanimación cardiopulmonar | |
| SAED (Semi-automatic External Defibrillator), DESA (Desfibrilador Externo Semiautomático) | |
| Heimlich Maneuver, maniobra de Heimlich | |
| mouth to mouth rescucitation, respiración boca a boca | |
| recovery position, PLS (posición lateral de seguridad) | |

# FIRST AID HEART ATTACK
# PRIMEROS AUXILIOS ATAQUE DE CORAZON

Heart attack, Los sintomas de un infarto

Women, En mujeres

Men, En hombres

- dizziness, mareos
- jaw pain, dolor de mandíbula
- throat discomfort, malestar en la garganta
- diarrhea, diarrea

Common symptoms, Sintomas comunes

- cold sweats, sudores fríos
- nausea, náuseas
- back pain, dolor de espalda

- neck pain, dolor en el cuello
- difficulty breathing, dificultad para respirar
- chest pain, dolor en el pecho
- pain in the left arm, dolor en el brazo izquierdo

# FIRST AID CHOKING- ASPHYXIA  PRIMEROS AUXILIOS -ATRAGAMIENTO -ASFIXIA

Signs of choking/airway obstruction, Signos de atragamiento/asfixia

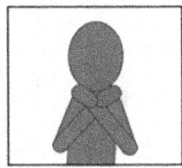

the universal sign of chocking
el signo universal de atragamiento

The signs of choking: Los signos de atragamiento:

·Face is bright red or blue. Cara de color rojo brillante o azulado.

·Grabs his or her throat. Agarrarse la garganta.

·Unable to cough strongly. No poder toser fuertemente.

·Difficulty speaking. Dificultad para hablar.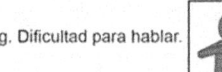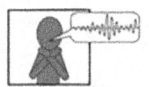

·Wheezing or a whistling sound. Resollar o un sonido silbante cuando trata de respirar.

# TYPES OF BURNS / TIPOS DE QUEMADURAS

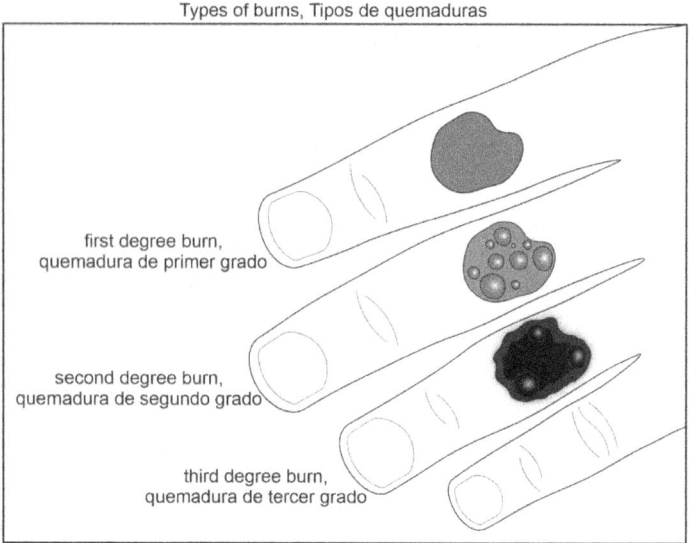

Types of burns, Tipos de quemaduras

first degree burn, quemadura de primer grado

second degree burn, quemadura de segundo grado

third degree burn, quemadura de tercer grado

# First Aid- Wounds / Primeros Auxilios-Heridas

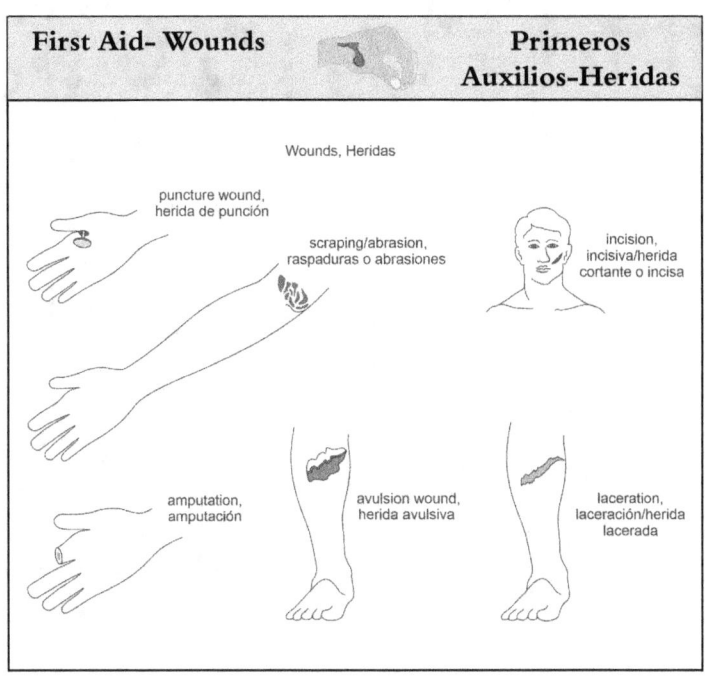

Wounds, Heridas

puncture wound, herida de punción

scraping/abrasion, raspaduras o abrasiones

incision, incisiva/herida cortante o incisa

amputation, amputación

avulsion wound, herida avulsiva

laceration, laceración/herida lacerada

# First Aid – hemorrhages 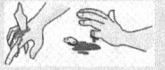 Primero Auxilios – hemorragias

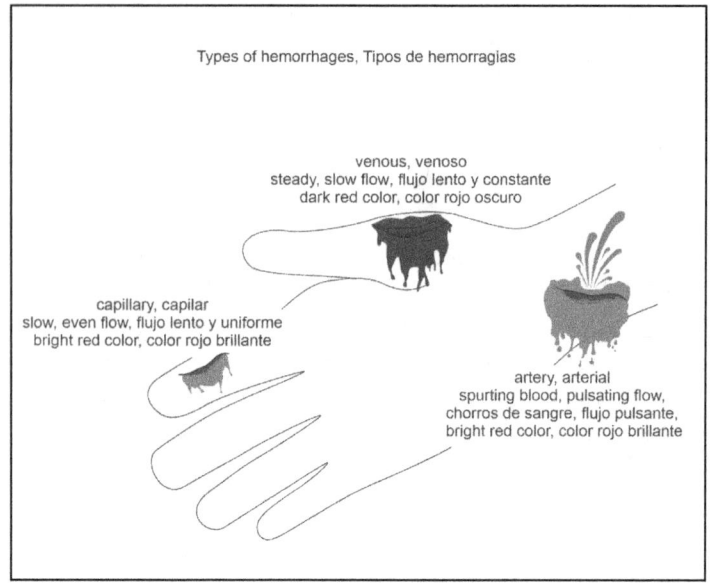

Types of hemorrhages, Tipos de hemorragias

venous, venoso
steady, slow flow, flujo lento y constante
dark red color, color rojo oscuro

capillary, capilar
slow, even flow, flujo lento y uniforme
bright red color, color rojo brillante

artery, arterial
spurting blood, pulsating flow,
chorros de sangre, flujo pulsante,
bright red color, color rojo brillante

# First Aid-Fractures  Primeros Auxilios-fracturas

Bone fractures,
Fracturas de hueso

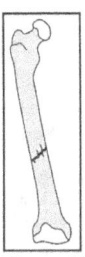
oblique, oblicua

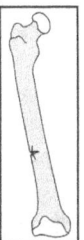
greenstick,
en tallo verde

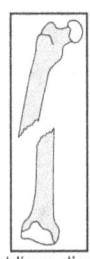
oblique displaced,
oblicuo desplazado

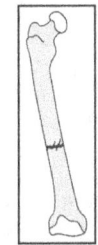
transverse, transversa

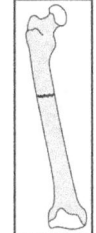
simple, simple

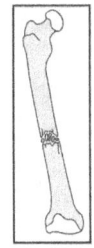
comminuted,
conminuta

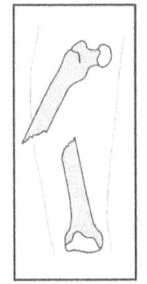
compound, compuesta

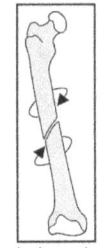
spiral, espiral

## Cardiology / Cardiología

The heart, El corazón

- aorta, arteria aorta
- superior vena cava, vena cava superior
- pulmonary artery, arteria pulmonar
- left atrium, aurícula izquierda
- pulmonary veins, venas pulmonares
- right atrium, aurícula derecha
- pulmonary veins, venas pulmonares
- valves, válvulas
- valves, válvulas
- right ventricle, ventrículo derecho
- left ventricle, ventrículo izquierdo
- inferior vena cava, vena cava inferior
- descending aorta, aorta descendente

## Heart diseases, Enfermedades cardíacas

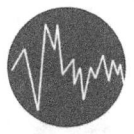 arythmia, arritmias

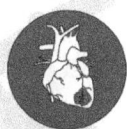 heart attack, ataque cardíaco

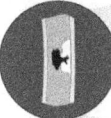 angina, anginas

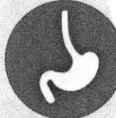 heart burn, acidez

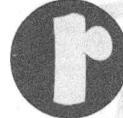 aneurism, aneurisma

 high cholesterol, colesterol alto

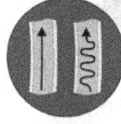 hypertension, hipertensión (high blood pressure) (presión arterial alta)

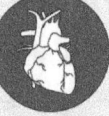 heart failure, paro cardiorespiratorio

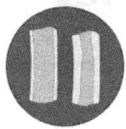 arteriosclerosis, arteroesclerosis

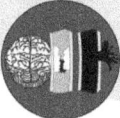 stroke, infarto/derrame cerebral

## Endocronology & Diabetes
## Endocrinología y diabetes

Endocrine system, Sistema endocrino

- hypothalamus, hipotálamo
- pituitary gland, glándula pituitaria
- thyroid gland, glándula tiroidea
- thymus gland, glándula timo
- adrenal glands (one on each kidney), glándulas suprarrenales (una en cada riñón)
- ovaries in females, ovarios en las mujeres
- glándula pineal, pineal gland
- parathyroid glands (on the posterior surface of the thyroid), glándulas paratiroides (en la superficie posterior de la tiroides)
- pancreas, páncreas
- testes in males, testículos en los hombres

## SYMPTOMS OF DIABETES
## SINTOMAS DE DIABETES

| | | | | |
|---|---|---|---|---|
| increased thirst *polidipsia/ aumento de la sed* | excessive/ increased urination-*poliuira/aumento de la micción* | fatigue-*fatiga* | blurry vision-*visión borrosa* | red & inflammed gums-*encías rojas e inflamadas* |
| unexpected weight loss-*pérdida de peso inesperada* | excessive eating-*polifagia/ aumento del hambre* | wounds that heal slowly-*llagas de curación lenta* | frequent infections-*infecciones frecuentes* | numbness or tingling in the hands or legs-*hormigueo o entumecimiento en las manos o los pies* |

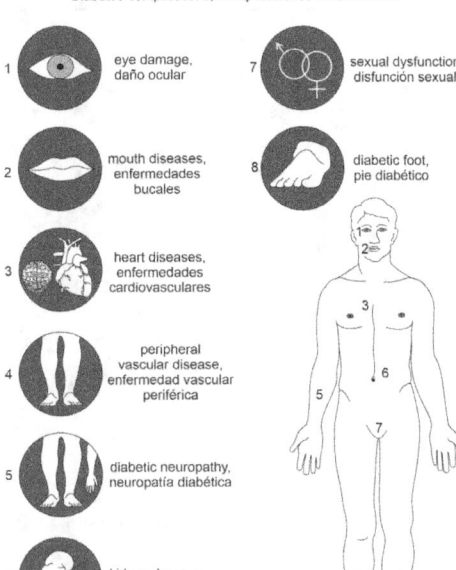

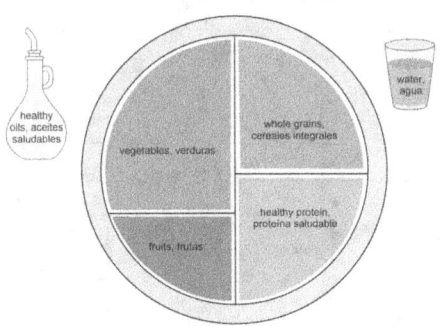

The healthy eating plate-created by Harvard Health Publishing and nutrition experts at the Harvard School of Public Health.
El plato para comer saludable- creado por expertos en nutrición de la Escuela de Salud Pública de Harvard y los editores en Publicaciones de Salud de Harvard.

# Oncology                             Oncología

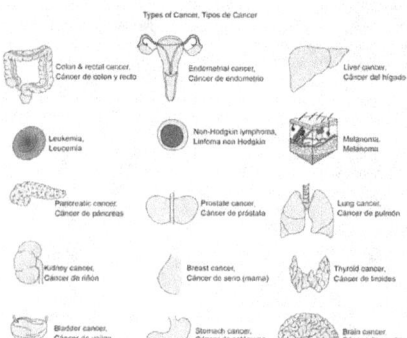

Types of Cancer, Tipos de Cáncer

- Colon & rectal cancer, Cáncer de colon y recto
- Endometrial cancer, Cáncer de endometrio
- Liver cancer, Cáncer del hígado
- Leukemia, Leucemia
- Non-Hodgkin lymphoma, Linfoma non Hodgkin
- Melanoma, Melanoma
- Pancreatic cancer, Cáncer de páncreas
- Prostate cancer, Cáncer de próstata
- Lung cancer, Cáncer de pulmón
- Kidney cancer, Cáncer de riñón
- Breast cancer, Cáncer de seno (mama)
- Thyroid cancer, Cáncer de tiroides
- Bladder cancer, Cáncer de vejiga
- Stomach cancer, Cáncer de estómago
- Brain cancer, Cáncer de cerebro

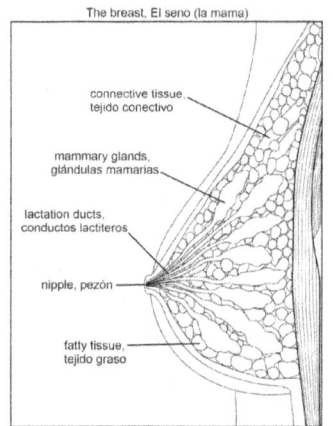

The breast, El seno (la mama)

- connective tissue, tejido conectivo
- mammary glands, glándulas mamarias
- lactation ducts, conductos lactíteros
- nipple, pezón
- fatty tissue, tejido graso

| Breast cancer symptoms | | | Síntomas del cáncer de mama | | |
|---|---|---|---|---|---|
| lump-bulto | swelling-hinchazón | dimple-hoyuelo | reddish area-área rojiza or enrojecimiento | nipple secretion-secreción por el pezón | pain in any part of the breast-dolor en cualquier parte de la mama |

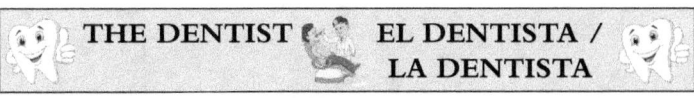

# THE DENTIST / EL DENTISTA / LA DENTISTA

Tooth anatomy, Anatomía del diente

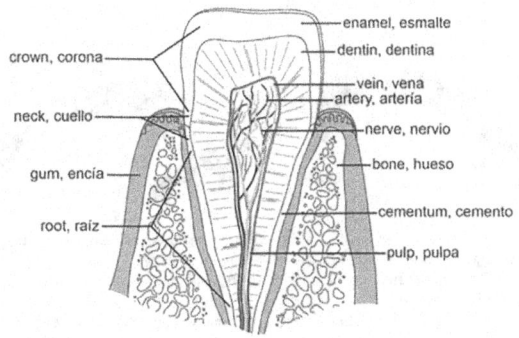

The teeth, Los dientes

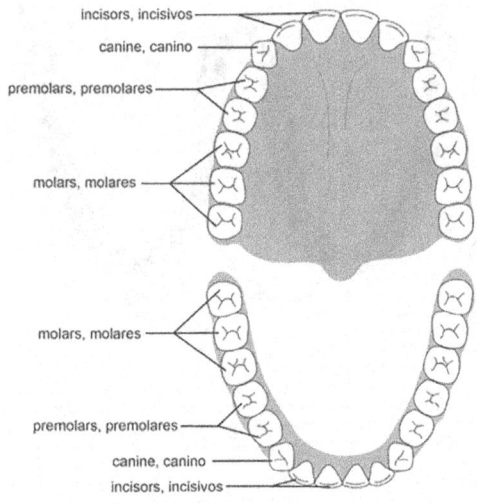

**Dental Initial Consultation** — **Consulta inicial con el dentista**

When was your last dental appointment? ¿Cuándo fue su última cita dental?
Who was your last dentist? ¿Quién fue su previo dentista?
When was the last time you saw a dentist? ¿Cuándo fue su última cita con el dentista?
Are you having any dental problems? ¿Está teniendo algún problema dental?
We are going to...... Vamos a ......
 take x-rays  tomar radiografías
 clean your teeth  limpiar sus dientes
 do an oral exam  hacer un examen oral
You have __ cavities. Ud tiene _____ caries.
How many times a day do you brush your teeth? ¿Cuántas veces al día se cepilla los dientes?
Do you use dental floss? ¿Usa hilo dental?

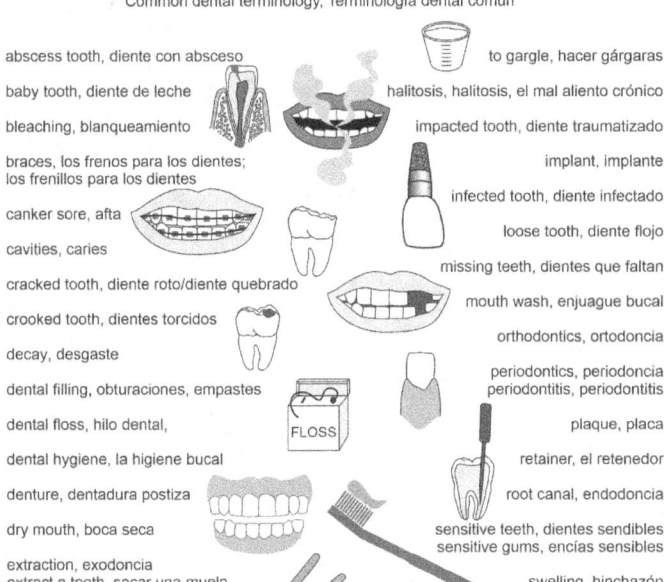

Common dental terminology, Terminología dental común

- abscess tooth, diente con absceso
- baby tooth, diente de leche
- bleaching, blanqueamiento
- braces, los frenos para los dientes; los frenillos para los dientes
- canker sore, afta
- cavities, caries
- cracked tooth, diente roto/diente quebrado
- crooked tooth, dientes torcidos
- decay, desgaste
- dental filling, obturaciones, empastes
- dental floss, hilo dental
- dental hygiene, la higiene bucal
- denture, dentadura postiza
- dry mouth, boca seca
- extraction, exodoncia
- extract a tooth, sacar una muela
- extruding tooth, diente extruído
- intruding tooth, diente intruído
- fluorid, flúor-florización
- to gargle, hacer gárgaras
- halitosis, halitosis, el mal aliento crónico
- impacted tooth, diente traumatizado
- implant, implante
- infected tooth, diente infectado
- loose tooth, diente flojo
- missing teeth, dientes que faltan
- mouth wash, enjuague bucal
- orthodontics, ortodoncia
- periodontics, periodoncia
- periodontitis, periodontitis
- plaque, placa
- retainer, el retenedor
- root canal, endodoncia
- sensitive teeth, dientes sendibles
- sensitive gums, encías sensibles
- swelling, hinchazón
- to brush one's teeth, cepillarse los dientes
- tooth ache, dolor de muelas
- tooth cleaning, limpieza dental

*take note* The American Dental Association (ADA) offers various resources in Spanish: MouthHealthy: MouthHealthy.org, a website both in English & Spanish that provides oral health information, **ADA Catalog: Patient education** brochures and books. The Hispanic Dental Association (HDA), offers !Sonrisa!, a free guide to dental health for Hispanic Americans. **American Association of Oral and Maxillofacial Surgeons** offers Spanish language patient information pamphlets.

| The Eyes –los ojos | 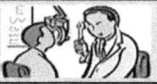 | The Eye Doctor –El ocultista |

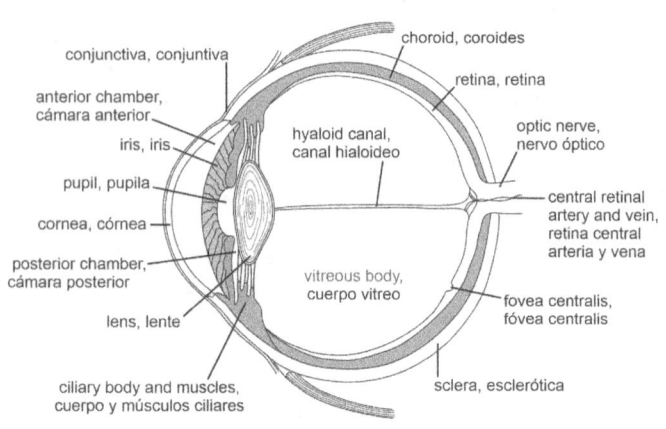

**Key eye phrases**

How is your vision? ¿Cómo está su vista?
Are there eye problems in your family? ¿Hay problemas de los ojos en su familia?
Do you have pain in your eye? Which eye? ¿Tiene dolor en su ojo? ¿Qúe ojo?
What drops do you use? ¿Que gotas usa?
Do you have any other eye sickness? ¿Tiene alguna enfermedad de los ojos?
Do you have any previous eye surgeries? ¿Tiene cirugias oculares previas?
Your eyes are healthy. Sus ojos son estables/sanos.
I'm going to give you an eyeglass prescription. Voy a darle una receta para lentes
I have to do surgery in your eye. Tengo que hacer cirugia en su ojo.

You need an eye examination. Necesita un examen de vista.
Eye Directions to Patient
Look here. Mire aquí, por favor.
Look ahead/up/down. Mire frente/ arriba/abajo.
Look left/right. Mire izquierda/derecha.
Open your eyes. Abra los ojos.
Close your eyes. Cierre los ojos.
Blink. íParpadee!

**EYE DISEASES**
astigmatism-astigmatismo
blind-ciego
cataract-catarata
color blindness-daltonismo
cross-eyed-bizco
glaucoma-glaucoma

**EYE COMPLAINTS**
blurry-borroso, nublado
floating spots-manchas flotantes
itchy- picante
burning-ardor
dry-seco
double-vision-vista doble

# DERMATOLOGY  DERMATOLOGIA

Skin, La piel

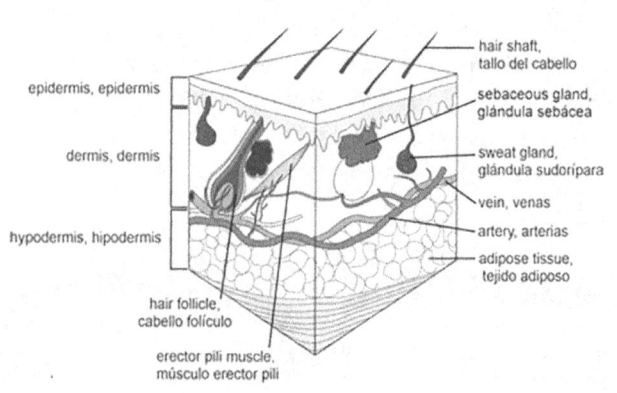

Types of skin cancer, Tipos de cáncer de la piel

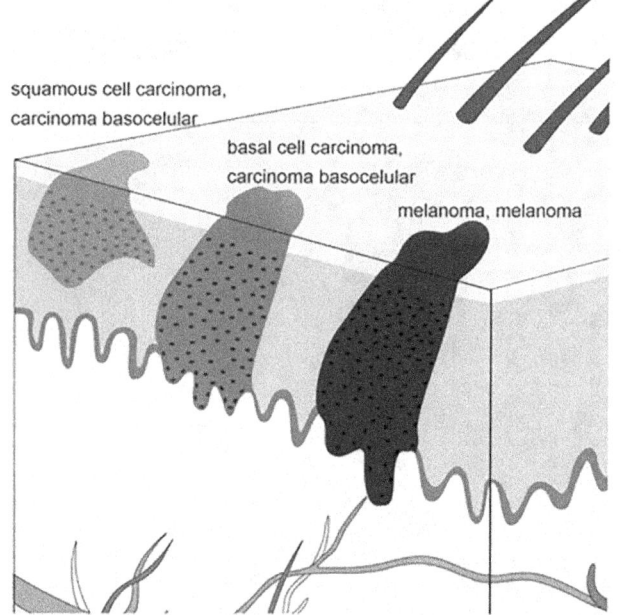

Medical dermatology - Dermatología médica

 acne, acné

 actinic keratosis, queratosis actínica

 blistering diseases of the skin, enfermedades ampollosas

 hair loss, pérdida del cabello

 urticaria, urticaria

 melanoma, melanoma

 moles and warts, lunares y verrugas

 nail fungus hongo de uñas

 skin pigmentation disorders, trastornos de la pigmentación

 scars, cicatrices

 skin allergies, alergias cutáneas

 skin cancer, cáncer de piel

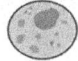 sun damage, daño del sol/daño solar

Skin problems, Problemas en la piel

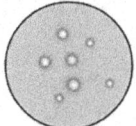
Acne, acné

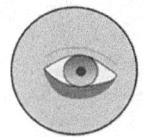
Dark circles, círculos oscuros debajo de los ojos

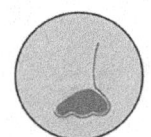
Redness, enrojecimiento de la piel

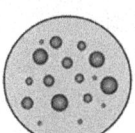
Clogged pores, poros obstruídos

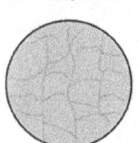
Dry/oily/normal skin, piel seca/grasa normal

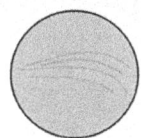
Wrinkles, arrugas

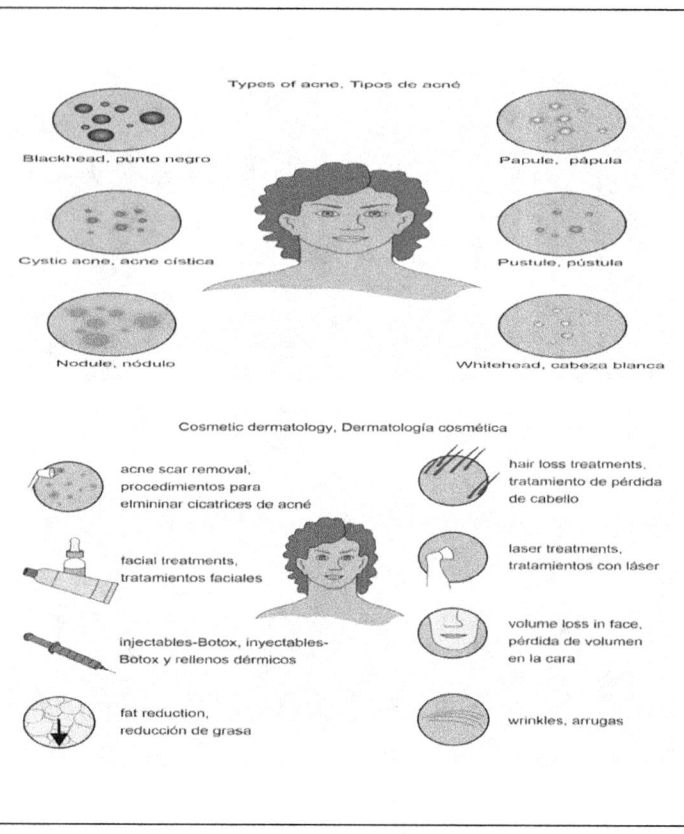

# ANATOMY SECTION  LOS SISTEMAS DEL CUERPO HUMANO

The head, La cabeza

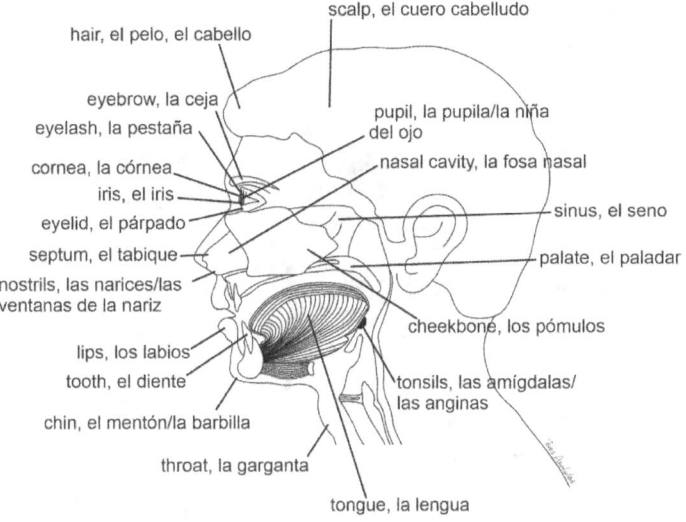

# THE MOUTH-LA BOCA

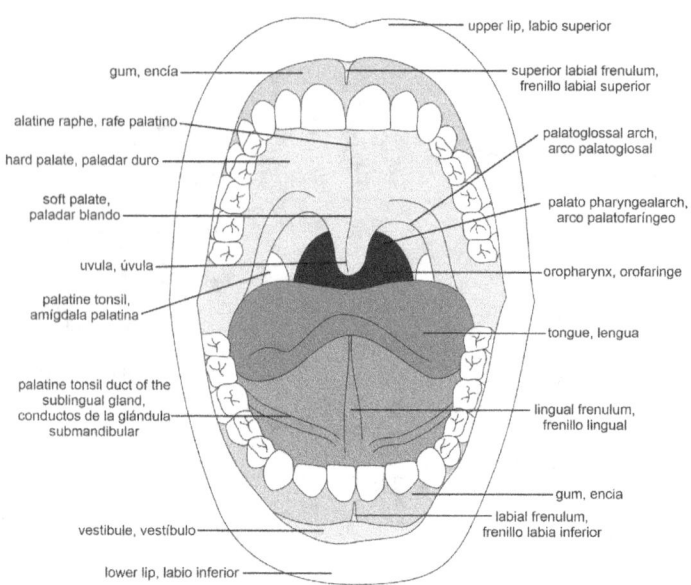

Mouth, Boca

# THE HUMAN BODY-EL CUERPO HUMANO

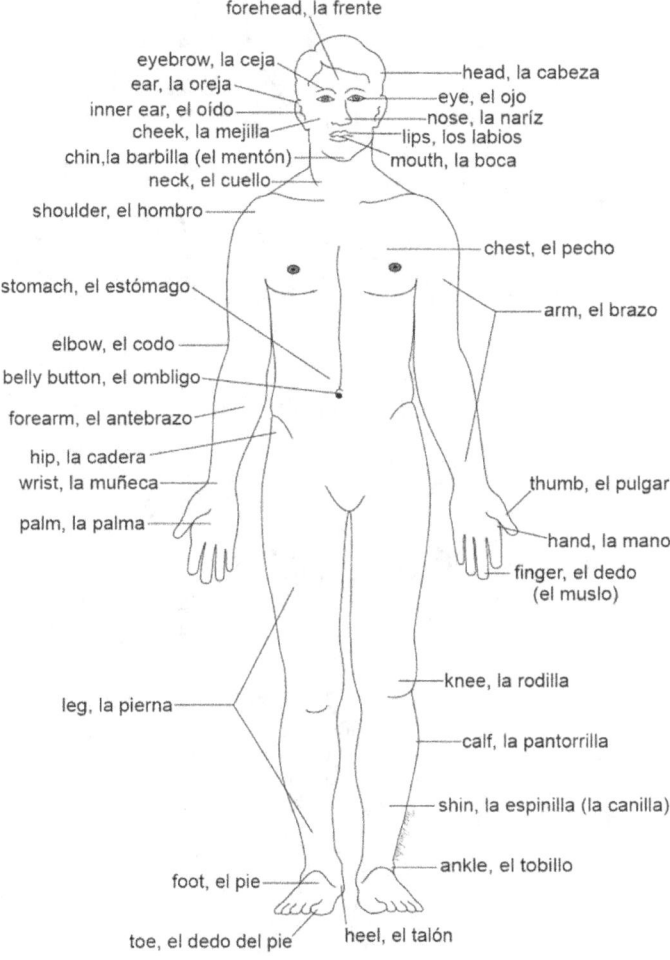

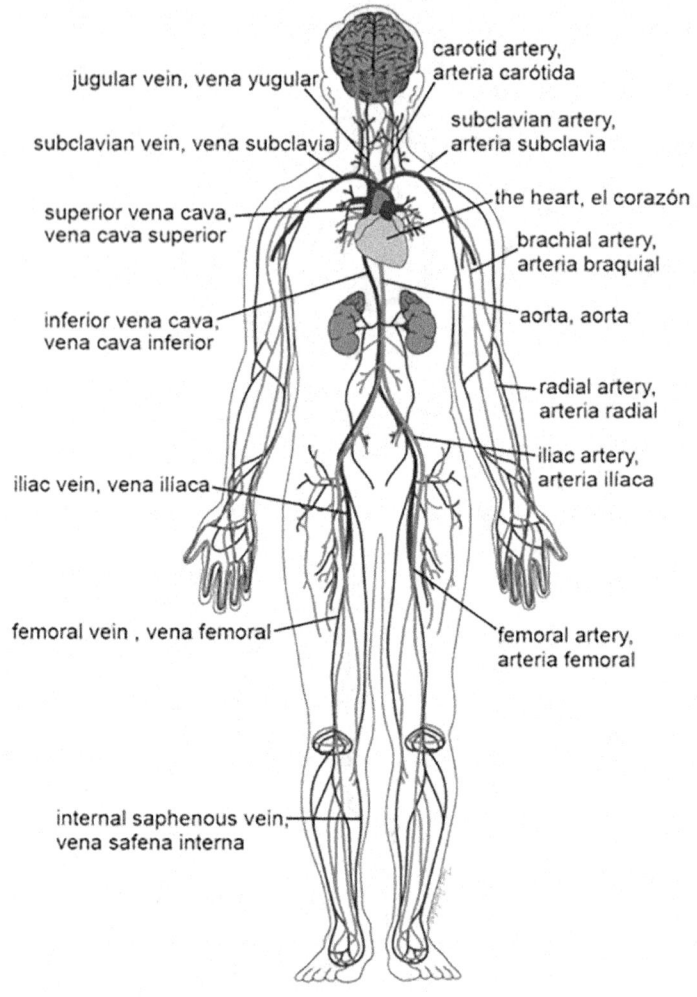

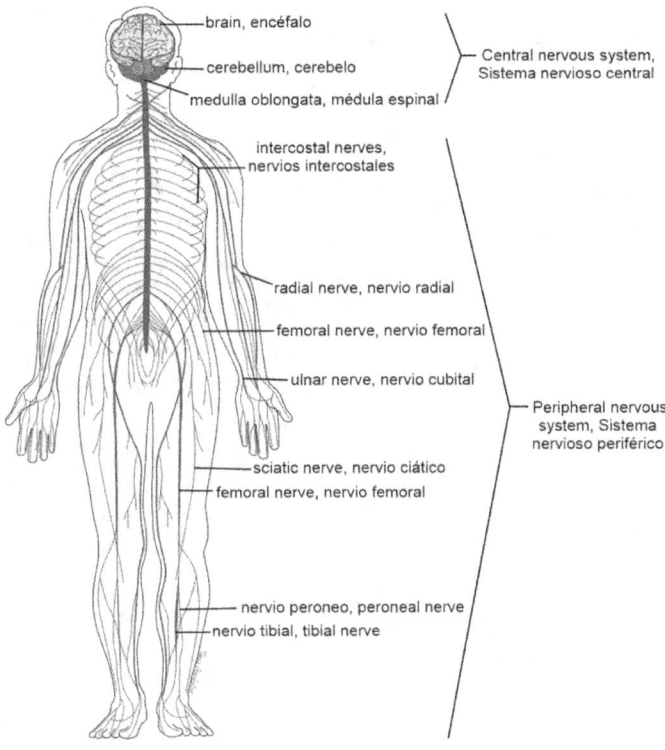

## Digestive system, Aparato digestivo

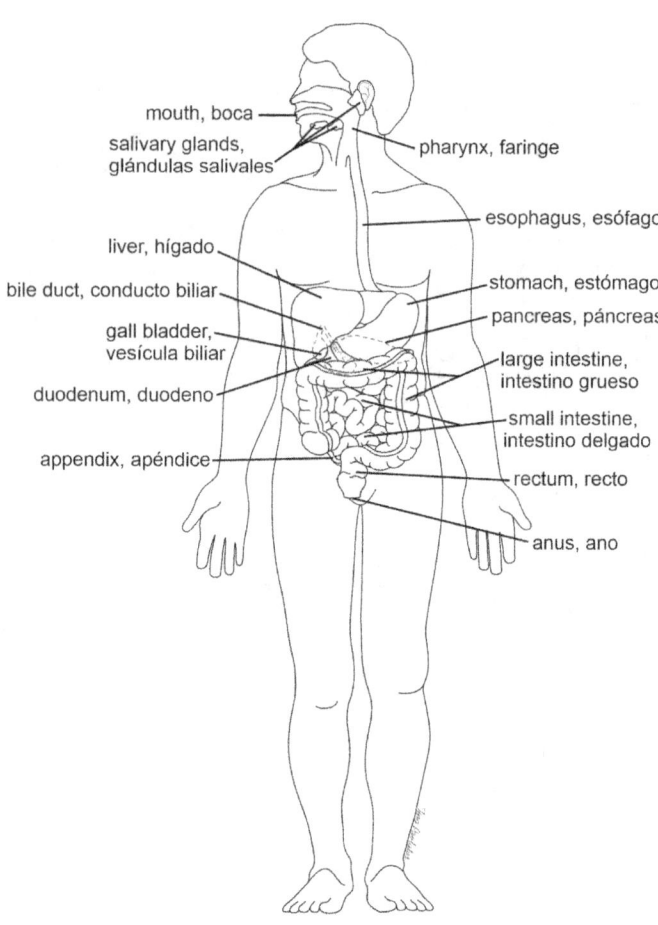

The respiratory system, El sisterna respiratorio

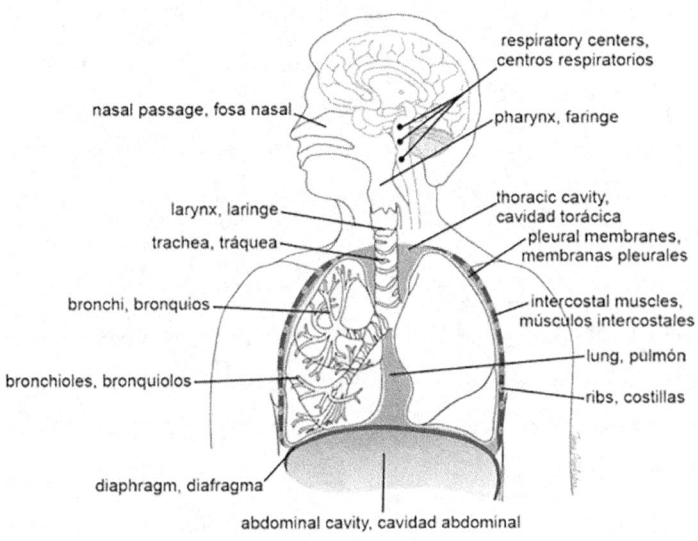

The skeletal system, El sistema esquelético,
(el sistema óseo)

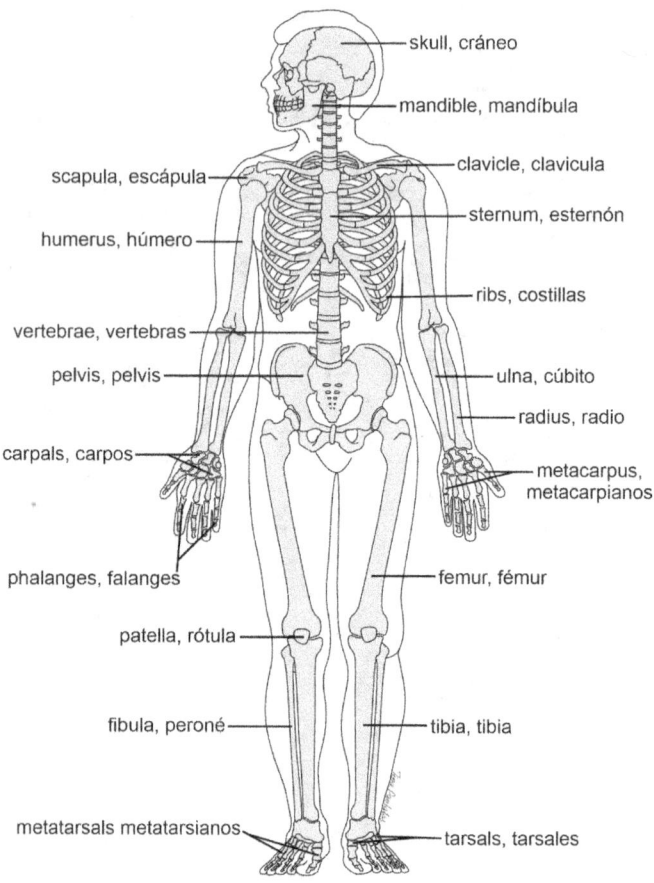

The muscular system, El sistema muscular

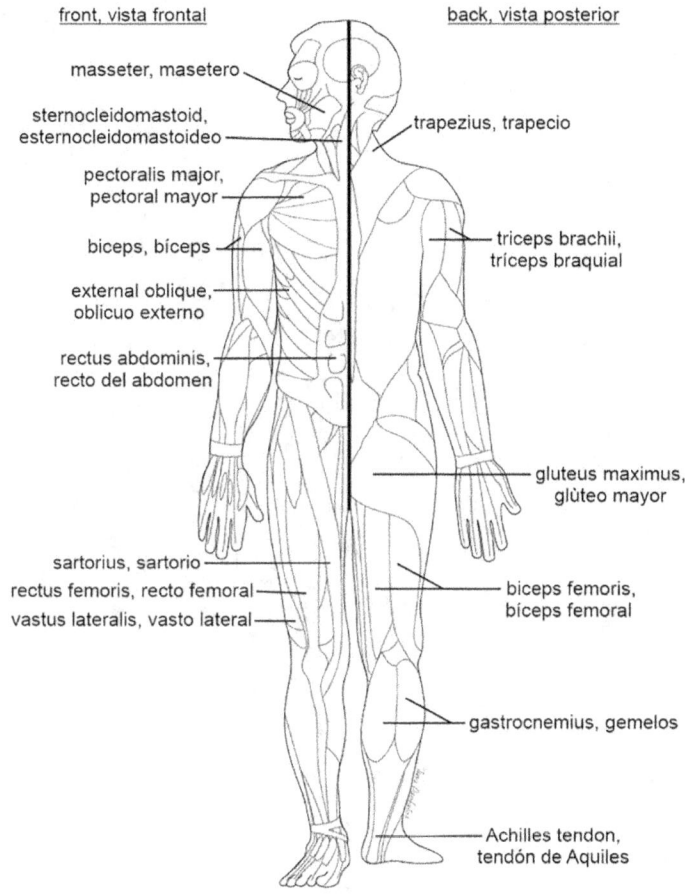

## The reproductive system, El sistema reproductor,

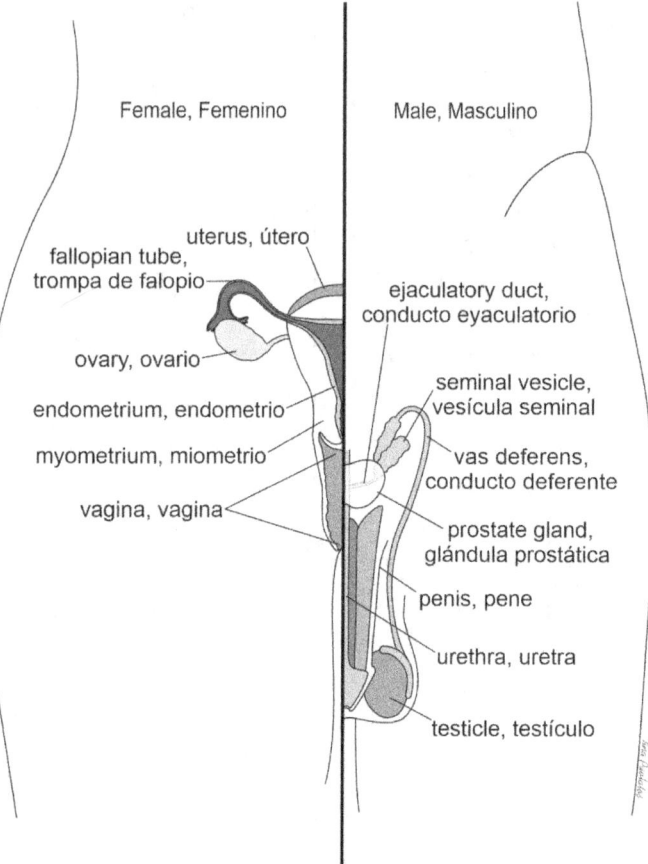

# BASIC CONVERSATION &  GRAMMAR SECTION

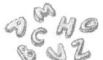
Alfabeto

Alphabet in Spanish, El Abecedario (Alfabeto)

| Letter | Letter Name | Pronunciation | Example |
|---|---|---|---|
| A | a | Sounds like the English *ah* | ambulancia |
| B | be (also called be larga, be grande or be de burro) | Often sounds like the English *b*. When between 2 vowels, it is pronounced much like the Spanish *v* (lips not touching) | biopsia |
| C | ce | Sounds like an English *s* if followed by a soft vowel (e or i ). Sounds like an English *k*, if followed by a consonant or a hard vowel (a, o, u) | cirugía camilla |
| CH | che | Sounds like an English *ch*; no longer considered a letter by RAE | chata |
| D | de | Sounds much like the English *d*. It is usually a softer sound, like *th* in English, especially when between 2 vowels | doctor |
| E | e | Sounds like *eh* in English | emergencia |
| F | efe | Sounds like an English *f* | fiebre |
| G | ge | Sounds like an English *g*, if followed by a consonant or a hard vowel (a, o,u); sounds like a harsh h if followed by a soft vowel (e or i ). | ginecólogo gaza |
| H | hache | As a general rule, this letter is silent if it is the first letter of a word. The exception to this rule are words adopted from other languages, which maintain the breathy aspiration, such as Hawáii. | hospital |
| I | i | Sounds like *ee* in English, but shorter | insulina |
| J | jota | Sounds like *h* in English | jeringa |
| K | ca | Sounds like *k* in English. The letter K is not native to the Spanish language & only appears in loanwords such as karate, kilo | kilómetro |
| L | ele | Sounds like the English *l*, (tongue raised closer to the roof of the mouth; not dipped) | laringitis |
| LL | doble ele | Sounds like 'y' in English (no longer considered a letter by RAE) | llaga |

| | | | |
|---|---|---|---|
| M | eme | Sounds like the English *m* | mamografía |
| N | ene | Sounds like the English *n* | neurología |
| Ñ | eñe | Sounds like the *ni* in onion or the *ny* in canyon | riñon |
| O | o | Sounds like the *o* in *so*, but shorter | operación |
| P | pe | Sounds like an English *p* | paperas |
| Q | cu | Always followed by a *u* and sounds like the English *k* | quemadura |
| R | erre | Sounds like the English *r*, but is rolled | rodilla |
| RR | doble erre | Trilled *rr* sound. No longer considered a letter by the RAE | socorro HELP! |
| S | ese | Sounds like an English *s* | sarampión |
| T | te | Sounds like an English *t but softer* | tos |
| U | u | Sounds like *oo* in *food* (note that when u is part of dipthong such as ua or ue, it sounds like an English *W*) | urólogo |
| V | ve or uve; also called ve corta, ve chica, ve de vaca | Sounds like the Spanish *b* (The lips don't touch and there is less aspiration) | vacuna |
| W | doble ve or uve doble | The letter *W* is not native to the Spanish language, but sounds like the English *w* & only appears in loanwords such as web & watt | síndrome de Down's |
| X | equis | Sounds like *ks* in English 'socks' | rayo X |
| Y | ye; also called I griega | Sounds like the *y* in English *yes*. At the end of a words, it sounds like the letter *I (hay)* | yodo |
| Z | zeta | Sounds like the Englsih *s*; in many parts of Spain it is a *th* sound | zumbido |

La Real Academia Española (RAE) or Royal Spanish Academy states that the Spanish alphabet has 27 letters. The Spanish language coincides with the English alphabet except that the Spanish alphabet has one additional letter, ñ (In 2010 RAE eliminated CH and LL as letters in Spanish alphabet).

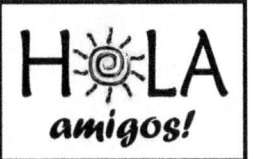

| Greetings & Good-byes 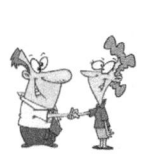 | Saludos y despedidas |
|---|---|
| Hello | Hola |
| Good morning | Buenos días |
| Good afternoon | Buenas tardes |
| Good evening | Buenas noches |
| Until... | Hasta + specific future time frame Example: Until next week. Hasta la semana próxima. |
| See you later | Hasta luego |
| See you tomorrow | Hasta mañana |
| See you soon | Hasta pronto or Hasta la vista |
| Have a nice day! | Que tenga un buen día |
| Goodbye | Adiós/Chau |

| Basic Daily Expressions  | Expresiones diarias |
|---|---|
| What's happening? | ¿Qué tal? ¿Qué pasa? |
| What's new? What's up? | ¿Qué hay de nuevo? |
| How's it going? (formal) | ¿Cómo le va? |
| How's it going? (familiar) | ¿Cómo te va? |

| Name  | Nombre |
|---|---|
| What is your name/last name? (formal) | ¿Cómo se llama? ¿Cuál es su nombre/apellido? |
| What is your name/last name? (familiar) | ¿Cómo te llamas? ¿Cuál es tu nombre/apellido? |

## Introductions
### Introducing yourself
## Presentaciones

My name is ...

Me llamo _____

Yo soy _____

Mi nombre es _____

### Introducing Others

I would like to introduce you to....

Le presento a...(formal)

Te presento a.. (familiar)

Nice to meet you.                    Mucho gusto.
It's a pleasure to meet you. (formal)    Es un placer conocerle.
It's a pleasure to meet you. (familiar)  Es un placer conocerte.
My pleasure.                         El placer es mío.
Charmed.                             Encantado/a

---

## Nationality / Nacionalidad

Where are you from ? (formal)       ¿De dónde es Usted?
Where are you from ? (familiar)     ¿De dónde eres tú?
I am from_____.                 Yo soy de_____.(country)

Yo soy_____(nationality)

**OJO take note:** Rules of Thumb for expressing nationality:

- Countries are capitalized. Nationalities are not capitalized. Example: I am from Mexico. Yo soy de México. I am Mexican. Yo soy mexicano/a.
- Adjectives of nationality must agree in gender and number with the noun they are referring to. They come after the noun. Example: la comida española (the Spanish food), el restaurante italiano (the Italian restaurant).
- The typical endings for adjectives of nationality in Spanish are: -ano, -ense, -l, -és, -eño, and -o. If the nationality ending is a consonant, add an –a for the feminine version.

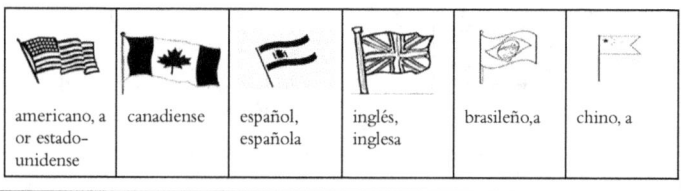

| americano, a or estado-unidense | canadiense | español, española | inglés, inglesa | brasileño, a | chino, a |
|---|---|---|---|---|---|

## Address — Dirección

Where do you live? (formal)     ¿Dónde vive Usted?
Where do you live? (familiar)     ¿Dónde vives?
I live in_____     Yo vivo en _____

## Profession/Job — Profesión/trabajo

What do you do? (formal)     ¿En qué trabaja? ¿En qué se dedica?
What do you do? (familiar)     ¿En qué trabajas? ¿En qué te dedicas?
I am a _____     Yo soy _____

**OJO** take note : To express someone's line of work use: SER + occupation or job. The article is omitted, unless you are adding an adjective to describe the person.
Example: I am a doctor. Yo soy médico,a. I am a kind doctor. Yo soy un médico amable.

## Health — Salud

How are you? (formal)     ¿Cómo está Usted?
How are you? (familiar)     ¿Cómo estás tú?
I am well .. sick ..regular ..so so     Estoy bien..enfermo(a) ....regular.. así así

## Looks & Personality Traits — Razcos físicos y razcos de la personalidad

What are you like? (formal)     ¿Cómo es Usted?
What are you like? (familiar)     ¿Cómo eres tú?
I am _____     Yo soy _____

**OJO** take note : Use the verb ser to describe essential qualities or intrinsic characteristics of a person or a thing, such as physical appearance and personality traits.
Example: Juan is tall, handsome and nice. Juan es alto, guapo y simpático.
Ana is blond, pretty and hard-working. Ana es rubia, bonita y trabajadora.

## Age  Edad

How old are you ? ¿Cúantos años tiene Usted ? (formal)

¿Cúantos años tienes tú ? (familiar)

I am _____ old. Yo tengo ___ años

**OJO** take note : Age is expressed with the verb tener in Spanish. It is one of the many idiomatic expressions with tener. Example: I am 20 years old. Yo tengo veinte años.

## Expressions of Courtesy    *Expresiones de cortesía*

| | |
|---|---|
| Thank you | Gracias |
| Please | Por favor |
| You're welcome | De nada |
| I'm sorry | Lo siento. |
| Pardon me | Perdón |
| Excuse me | Disculpe or Con permiso. |
| Take care | Cuídese (formal) Cuídate (familiar). |
| Bless you! | ¡Salud! (after someone sneezes) |
| Welcome! | ¡Bienvenido(a)! |

# Telling Time in Spanish

What time is it?   ¿Qué hora es?

OJO **take note**: ¿Qué hora es? Literally means What hour is it? When telling time in Spanish, the word hour (hora) is implied.

## To tell time in Spanish:

Es la \_\_\_\_. Use for 1:00 o'clock (am or pm). Example: It is 1:00 o'clock. Es la una.

Son las _____. Use for any hour greater than 1:00am or pm. Example: It is 8:00 o'clock. Son las ocho. It is 2:00 o'clock. Son las dos.

**OJO:** *take note* The feminine article (*la/las*) is used before the number because it refers to la hora.

## ADDING OR SUBTRACTING MINUTES:

To add minutes: use 'y' which means 'and'. Example: It is 8:10. Son las ocho y diez.

To subtract minutes: use 'menos' which means 'less' or 'minus'. Example: It is 9:50. Son las diez menos diez.

To express 15 minutes: use 'cuarto' or 'quince'. Example: It is 5:15. Son las cinco y quince. OR Son las cinco y cuarto.

To express half an hour, use 'media'. Example: It is 10:30. Son las diez y media.

**OJO:** *take note* There are 2 ways to express time past the half hour:
a) Round up to the next hour after the half hour mark and subtract minutes. Example: It is 8:40. Son las nueve menos veinte.

OR

Express time numerically. Example: It is 8:40. Son las ocho y cuarenta.

To express time of day use:
- *mediodía* – midday
- *mañana* – in the morning
- *noche* – at night
- *madrugada* – the middle of the night
- *medianoche* – midnight
- *amanecer* – dawn
- *tarde* – in the afternoon

Rules for specifying time of day (morning, afternoon or evening):

To express AM (if specifying an exact time): use 'de la mañana'
Example: It is 9:00am. Son las nueve de la mañana.

To express afternoon (if specifying an exact time): use 'de la tarde'.
Example: It is 4:00pm. Son las cuatro de la tarde.

To express PM: use 'de la noche' (if specifying an exact time):
Example: It is 9:00pm. Son las nueve de la noche.

**OJO:** If you are not specifying the time of day, use por la mañana (in the morning), por la tarde (in the afternoon) and por la noche (in the evening).

Example:
I work in the morning. Yo trabajo por la mañana.
Juan goes to the gym in the afternoon. Juan va al gimnasio por la tarde.
The students study in the evening. Los estudiantes estudian por la noche.

# Expressing Dates in Spanish

What is today's date? ¿Cuál es la fecha de hoy?

| Day of week los días de la semana | | | | | | |
|---|---|---|---|---|---|---|
| Monday | Tuesday | Wesnesday | Thursday | Friday | Saturday | Sunday |
| lunes | martes | miércoles | jueves | viernes | sábado | domingo |

OJO take note Days of the week in Spanish are lower case, masculine and are not pluralized except for Saturday & Sunday. The first day of the week is Monday.

## Months - Los meses

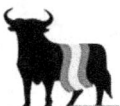

| January | February | March | April | May | June |
|---|---|---|---|---|---|
| enero | febrero | marzo | abril | mayo | junio |
| July | August | September | October | November | December |
| julio | agosto | septiembre | octubre | noviembre | diciembre |

OJO take note In Spanish, you will first say the day of the week, the number of the associated day, then the month followed by the year.

**Example: What is today's date? ¿Cuál es la fecha de hoy? Today is Monday, January 10, 2022. Hoy es lunes, el diez de enero de 2022.**

### Seasons & months 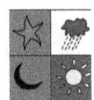 Estaciones y meses del año

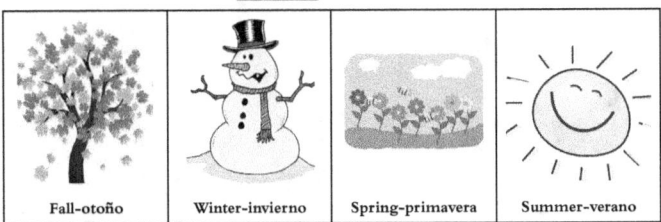

| Fall-otoño | Winter-invierno | Spring-primavera | Summer-verano |

# GENDER & NOUNS IN SPANISH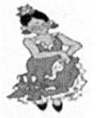

Every noun in Spanish is either masculine or feminine.

## BASIC GENDER RULES

| Masculine nouns end in: -O, -L, -N, -R, -S -Y, -PA, -MA, -TA, -AJE, -ZON<br>Examples: | Feminine nouns end in: -A, -D (-TAD, -TUD -DAD, -ED), -CION, -SION, -UMBRE<br>Examples: |
|---|---|
| ---O el libro | ---A la casa |
| ---L el árbol | ---TAD la libertad |
| ---N el camión | ---TUD gratitud |
| ---R el amor | ---DAD La ciudad - |
| ---S el país | ---ED la sed |
| ---Y el rey- | ---CION la conversación |
| ---PA el mapa | ---SION la televisión |
| ---MA el idioma | ---UMBRE muchedumbre |
| ---TA el planeta | |
| ---AJE el viaje | |
| ---ZON el corazón | |

**OJO** take note :There are exceptions to the above rules. Example: la mano-the hand, el día-the day. The gender of a noun (m. or f.) can be found next to the word in a Spanish dictionary. An excellent reference is the main Spanish dictionary, Diccionario de la Real Academia Española (DRAE),

Additional Gender Rules:

♀♀ **LIVING THINGS**  People or living creatures are referred to by the gender they represent. Example: the boy→ el chico, the girl→ la chica.

♀♀ **MIXED GENDER**  If you are referring to a group of people with mixed gender, you must always use the masculine, even if the ratio of males is less than the ratio of females. Example: los chicos (if a mix of male and female).

♀♀ **PROFESSIONS**  Profession nouns change to match the gender of the person they refer to. Many profession nouns have masculine forms that end in o. These nouns can be made feminine by changing the o to an a. Example: el médico→ the male doctor, la médica→ the female doctor.

**OJO** take note: There are some professions that keep the same form in the noun and change article only. Example: el piloto, la piloto.
**-ISTA** If a noun ends in –*ista* only the article changes to match the gender of the person.
Example: *el artista* → the male artist     *la artista* → the female artist.

♀♀ If the masculine of a noun endings in-r, the feminine will add an –a.
*Example: el director* → the male director *la directora* → the female director

♀♀ The article can change the meaning of a word.
Example: el cura → the priest     la cura → the cure

♀♀ Letters of the alphabet are feminine. Days of the week are masculine.

**OJO** : Nouns that do not refer to living creatures follow basic gender rules, regardless of whether they are typically associated with males or females. Example: el vestido 👗 la corbata 👔

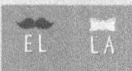 **The word THE is expressed 4 different ways in Spanish:**

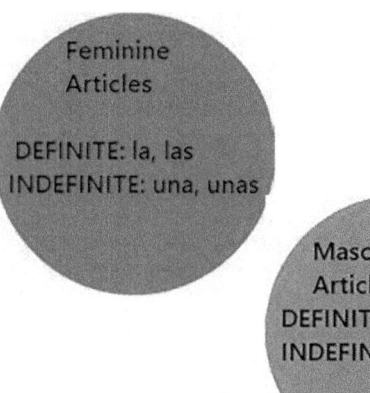

Feminine Articles

DEFINITE: la, las
INDEFINITE: una, unas

Masculine Articles
DEFINITE: el, los
INDEFINITE: un, unos

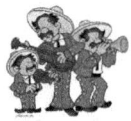 **PLURALS IN SPANISH**

| IF A NOUN ENDS IN A VOWEL: ADD –S | IF A NOUN ENDS IN A CONSONANT: ADD –ES |
|---|---|
| IF A NOUN ENDS IN A –Z: CHANGE TO -CES | **OJO** if a noun is plural, the adjective following it and the article preceding it must also be plurals |

**Possessives adjectives**

**Possessives adjectives show ownership. They are placed before a noun. Possessives adjectives agree in number to the noun. The nosotros & vosotros forms agree in gender as well.**

| PRONOUN | singular | plural | examples |
|---|---|---|---|
| my | mi | mis | mi sombrero<br>mis sombreros |
| your (familiar) | tu | tus | tu casa<br>tus casas |
| his, hers, your (formal), its | su | sus | su vestido<br>sus vestidos |
| our | nuestro, nuestra | nuestros, nuestras | nuestra manzana<br>nuestras manzanas<br>nuestro helado<br>nuestros helados |
| your (all) Spain | vuestro, vuestra | vuestros, vuestras | vuestro zapato<br>vuestros zapatos<br>vuestra corbata<br>vuestras corbatas |
| their, your (all) Latin America | su | sus | su hamburguesa<br>sus hamburguesas |

**OJO** take note 'Su' and 'sus' can mean his, hers, yours (formal) its, their or your (plural-Latin America). 'Su' should always be used when the noun is singular and 'sus' should always be used when the noun is plural. example: su casa or sus casas.

**RULE OF THUMB:** *'Su'* should always be used when the noun is singular and **'sus'** should always be used when the noun is plural. For clarification, use the possessive de. Example: *Es su libro* can be stated as *Es el libro de Juan*.

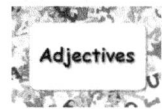

**OJO** take note Adjectives agree in gender and number with the noun they modify.

| angry | Happy | Bored | Nice |
|---|---|---|---|
| Enojado/a/os/as | Feliz/felices or Contento/a/os/as | Aburrido/a/os/as | Simpático/a/os/as |
| Mean/nasty | Smart | Beatiful-lindo/a/os/as  Pretty-bonito/a/os/as | Handsome |
| Antipático/a/os/as | Inteligente/s | | Guapo/a/o/os |
| Ugly | Fat | Skinny | Tall |
| Feo/a/os/as | Gordo/a/os/as | Delgado/a/os/as | Alto/a/os/as |

**OJO** take note: The rule of thumb regarding placement of nouns and adjectives is QUANTITY BEFORE QUALITY. Example: Ten intelligent nurses would be Diez enfermeras/os inteligentes. Adjectives follow the noun that they modify and agree in gender & in number with the noun that they modify.

**Demonstrative Adjectives**-denote distance of an object or person in relation to the speaker

| Distance from speaker | Masculine singular | Masculine plural | Feminine singular | Feminine plural |
|---|---|---|---|---|
| Close-this & these | **este** | **estos** | **esta** | **estas** |
| farther -that & those | **ese** | **esos** | **esa** | **esas** |
| Farthest-that & those | **aquel** | **aquellos** | **aquella** | **aquellas** |

**OJO** take note: If the noun **is not identified**, is **abstract, or is unknown**, the neuter demonstrative pronouns esto, eso, and aquello are used.

**Examples: Este libro. This book (CLOSEST TO THE SPEAKER)**

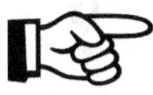 

**Ese libro. That book. (FURTHER FROM THE SPEAKER)**

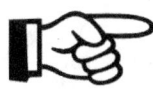 

**Aquel libro. That book over there. (FURTHEST FROM THE SPEAKER)**

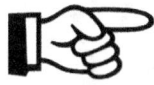 

**OJO** take note: EASY WAY TO REMEMBER: this & these have the 't's.

## QUESTION WORDS

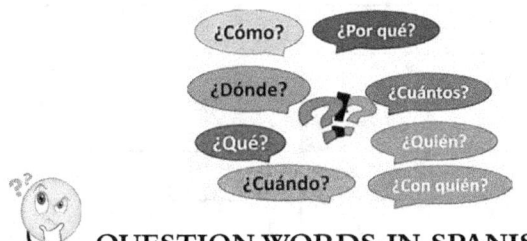

**QUESTION WORDS IN SPANISH**

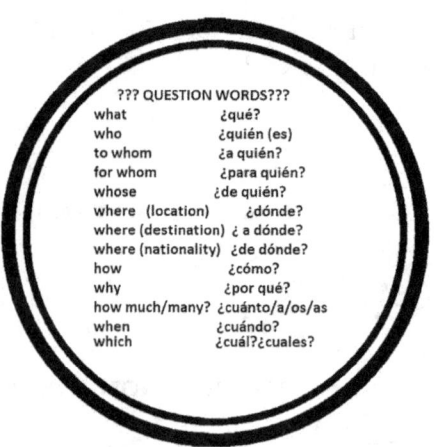

**OJO** take note There are 3 different variations of the question word 'dónde'. Use ¿Dónde? if you are inquiring about location of something or someone. Use ¿A dónde? if you are inquiring about a destination and use ¿De dónde? if you are inquiring about someone's nationality.

## SPANISH PRONOUN CHART

**OJO** take note Pronouns are key to mastering Spanish grammar. Below are 4 **MUST KNOW** types of pronouns in Spanish:

| Subject pronouns | Reflexive Pronouns | DOP | IDOP |
|---|---|---|---|
| Yo-I | me | me | me |
| Tú (you familiar) | te | te | te |
| Él, ella, Usted | se | lo, la | le |
| nosotros | nos | nos | nos |
| vosotros | os | os | os |
| Ellos, ellas, Uds | se | los, las | les |

# SUBJECT PRONOUNS

In Spanish, subject pronouns are generally used for emphasis or clarity. Unlike in English, in Spanish you can omit a personal pronoun before a verb. The verb conjugations make clear the subject of the sentence. For example: **Hablas español.** *You speak Spanish.* **Hablamos español.** *We speak Spanish.* The 3rd person singular or plural is where there is room for ambiguity because the 3rd person singular can be he, she, you (formal) or it.

**OJO** take note There is no equivalent translation for the subject pronoun "it". You simply omit the subject pronoun altogether and use the 3rd person of the verb: **Es bonita.** *It is beautiful.* **Funciona bien.** *It works well.*

| | |
|---|---|
| Yo – I | nosotros, as – we |
| Tú – you (familiar) | vosotros – you all (Spain) |
| él – he<br>ella – she<br>Usted (you formal) | ellos, ellas – they<br>Ustedes (you all Latin America) |

**OJO** take note **In Spanish there are two personal pronouns for "***you***" singular: tú and usted.**

**Tú** is used informally, i.e when talking to a friend, a person we know well, a child, young people and someone that you would address on a first-name basis.

**Usted** is used formally, i.e when talking to a person you do not know, someone who is older, or someone you are addressing with a title.

# Reflexive Pronouns

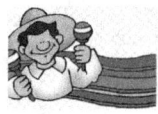

Reflexive verbs reflect back to the person doing the action. They are used only if the subject is doing the action to themselves.

The verb 'lavar' is an example of this concept. It can be used as lavar (non-reflexive) or lavarse (reflexive). The key is who is the subject doing the action to.

Example: I wash the car. Yo lavo el coche. (the subject does the action to the car) Juan washes the pet. Juan lava el mascote. (the subject does the action to the pet) Therefore, no reflexive is needed.

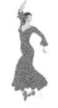

| NON REFLEXIVE | | REFLEXIVE | |
|---|---|---|---|
| Yo lavo | Nosotros lavamos | Yo me lavo | Nosotros nos lavamos |
| Tú lavas | Vosotros laváis | Tú te lavas | Vosotros os laváis |
| Él, ella, Ud lava | Ellos, ellas, Uds lavan | Él, ella, Usted Se lava | Ellos, ellas, Uds Se lavan |

EXAMPLES: I wash myself. Me lavo. Juan washes himself. Juan se lava. We wash ourselves. Nos lavamos. (The subject does the action to themselves).

**OJO** take note Some common reflexive verbs in Spanish are daily routine verbs such as despertarse (to wake up), bañarse- to take a bath, ducharse-to take a shower, maquillarse-to put on makeup, afeitarse- to shave.

**Direct & Indirect Object Pronouns**

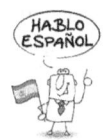

OJO *take note* To figure out which is the direct object and which is the indirect object of a sentence, your starting point is always the **subject and verb of the sentence**.

DOP (Direct Object Pronoun) —Answers the question '**who or what**' with regard to the verb. A DOP can be a person, place or thing. Ex. I read <u>the book</u>. I read it. Julia loves <u>Miguel</u>. Julia loves him

IDOP (Indirect Object Pronoun)-Aswers the question '**to whom, for whom**' with regard to the verb and is usually found at the end of the sentence. IDOPs always refer to a person. Example: Jorge buys the book <u>for Juan</u>. Jorge buys the book for him.

**DOP Rules of Thumb:**

In English the order is verb +DOP. In Spanish the order is DOP + verb for simple sentences (the rule changes when you have 2 verbs together)

Example: Juan lee <u>el libro</u>. Juan **lo** lee. Juan reads the book. Juan reads it.

**IDOP Rules of Thumb:**

In English the order is verb + IDOP. In Spanish, the order is IDOP + verb. (the rule changes when you have 2 verbs together)

Example: Juan reads the book to Geraldo. Juan **le** lee el libro.

OJO *take note* The 3rd person 'le' can mean to him, to her, to you (formal) or to it (such as a pet). You can use context to figure out who it is referring to or you add a clarifier to a sentence Example-

Yo **le** doy la computadora **a Jorge**. The clarifier ' a Jorge', lets the reader know that 'le' in this case, is to him or to Jorge.

**Direct & Indirect Object Pronouns TOGETHER**

In Spanish, as in English, you can use both DOPs & IDOPs in a sentence together .

**DOP & IDOP TOGETHER Rules of Thumb:**

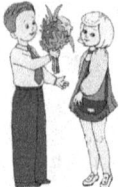

SPANISH: IDOP + DOP + verb (English: verb + DOP + IDOP)

DOP-answers the question 'what or who'

IDOP-answers the question 'to whom'

Juan gives flowers to me. Juan gives them to me.

Juan da las flores a mí. Juan me las da.

In English, the order for IDOP & DOPs used together is verb+DOP+IDOP. In Spanish the order is IDOP+DOP+verb for simple sentences (the rule changes when you have 2 verbs together).

Example. I read the book to you (familiar). I read it to you. Yo **te lo** leo.

OJO take note In Spanish you can never have an indirect and direct object that both start with an 'l'. You must substitute the indirect object with the pronoun 'se'. Example- Yo doy el libro a Juan. Yo le lo doy is incorrect. You must say: Yo se lo doy.

SPANISH: IDOP + DOP + verb (English: verb + DOP + IDOP)

DOP-answers the question 'what or who'

IDOP-answers the question 'to whom'

Juan gives flowers to Marta. Juan gives them to her.

Juan da las flores a Marta. Juan le las da IS INCORRECT. 'LE' becomes 'SE'. CORRECT ANSWER: Juan se las da.

|   VERBS –In Spanish there are 3 types of verbs: -ar, -er, -ir |
|---|

|  REGULAR VERB ENDINGS FOR –AR, -ER & -IR VERBS |
|---|

The subject or subject pronoun determines which ending to use.

| Subject Pronoun | Habl-ar | Com-er | Viv-ir |
|---|---|---|---|
| Yo | Habl-o | Com-o | Viv-o |
| Tú | Habl-as | Com-es | Viv-es |
| Él, ella, Usted | Habl-a | Com-e | Viv-e |
| Nosotros | Habl-amos | Com-emos | Viv-imos |
| Vosotros | Habl-áis | Com-éis | Viv-ís |
| Ellos, ellas, Ustedes | Habl-an | Com-en | Viv-en |

**OJO** *take note* Vosotros (you all-addressing a group of people) is used in Spain and Ustedes (you all-plural), is used in Latin America. You may hear a variation of vosotros in Argentina or Colombia, ex -Vos trabajás (you work).

# SER VS ESTAR – In Spanish, there are two verbs that mean 'to be'.

| ESTAR: yo estoy, tú estás, él, ella, Usted está, nosotros estamos, vosotros estáis, ellos están  | SER: yo soy, tú eres, él, ella, Ud es, nosotros somos vosotros sois ellos, ella, Uds son  |
|---|---|
| ESTAR-used for temporary, or changeable situations (acronym-HELP) | SER-used for situations considered permanent-(acronym DOCTOR) |
| H= health 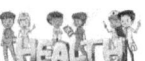<br><br>E = emotions or mood 😊😊😊😎😉😐😤😠😵 | DATE 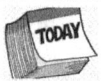 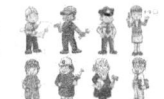<br><br>OCCUPATION |
| L=location  | CHARACTERISTIC (looks or intrinsic characteristic) 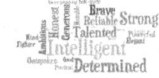 |
| P=present progressive or present temporary condition 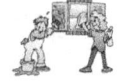 | TIME 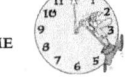 |
| PREPOSITIONS OF LOCATION USED WITH ESTAR 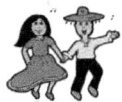 | ORIGIN (NATIONALITY) 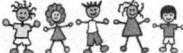 |
| OJO<br>USE ESTAR TO FORM THE PRESENT PROGRESSIVE<br>ESTAR + ando for –ar verbs<br>ESTAR + -iendo for –er & -ir verbs | RELATION (Relationships to someone, what something is made of & possession or ownership) 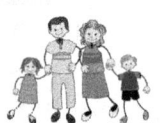 |

**OJO** take note Ser & estar both have different uses. They can not be interchanged without affecting the meaning.

| Ser aburrido/a | To be boring | Estar aburrido/a | To be bored |
|---|---|---|---|
| Ser listo/a | To be clever | Estar listo/a | To be ready |
| Ser orgulloso/a | To be conceited | Estar orgulloso/a | To be proud |
| Ser rico/a | To be rich | Estar rico/a | To be tasty |
| Ser seguro/a | To be safe | Estar seguro/a | To be certain |
| Ser malo | To be bad | Estar malo | To be ill |

# PREPOSITIONS OF LOCATION

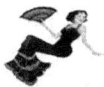

Prepositions of location are used to show the location of a person or an item usually in relation to something or someone else. They are used with the verb estar.

| *In front of* *Enfrente de, delante de* | *Next to Al lado de* | To the left *A la izquierda de* | To the right *A la derecha de* |
|---|---|---|---|
| Los libros están delante del chico. | El perro está al lado del hombre. | La niña está sentada a la izquierda del pupitre. | La niña está sentada a la derecha del pupitre. |
| Under *debajo de* La pelota está debajo de la mesa. | Around *Alrededor de* La familia está alrededor de la mesa. | *On/upon Sobre* Los libros están sobre la mesa. | Between *Entre* El plato está entre la cuchara y el tenedor. |
| Inside dentro de El niño está dento de la caja. | Behind *Detrás de* La pizarra está detrás del profesor. | Close to - *Cerca de* El hombre está cerca de la mujer. | Far from *Lejos de* El chico está lejos de la casa. |

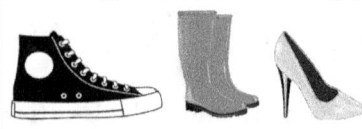

**STEM CHANGING VERBS** - also referred to as SHOE, BOOT, SNEAKER VERBS.

There are 4 different types: **o:ue, e:ie, e:i, u:ue (jugar-to play-is the only u:ue stem-changing verb)**.

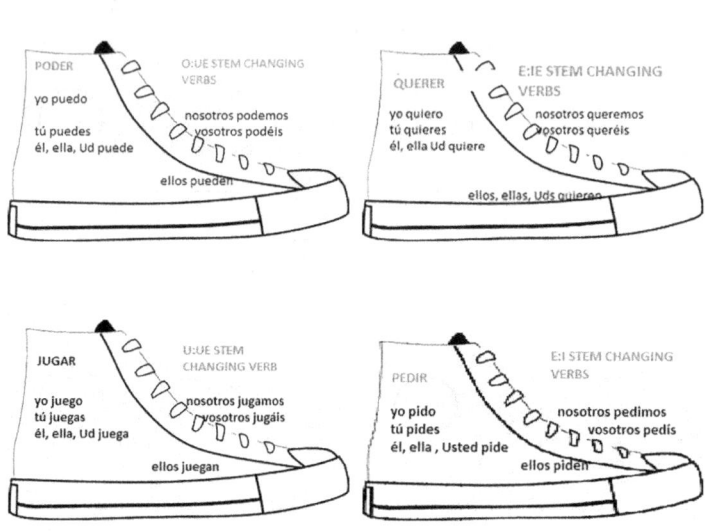

**OJO** take note The stem-changing verbs are classified as shoe/boot/sneaker verbs to facilitate learning their conjugations for the beginner student. Shoe verbs have stem changes in every form except nosotros & vosotros. They are classified as shoe verbs because both nosotros & vosotros are outside of the shoe. All regular forms are outside the shoe.

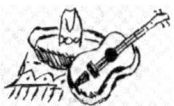

**GO VERBS** - Verbs that have a go ending in the yo form

## The Spanish "yo-go" verbs are as follows:

| decir (to say) **yo digo** | hacer (to do/make) **yo hago** | poner (to put) **yo pongo** | salir (to leave/**go** out) **yo salgo** |
|---|---|---|---|
| oir (to listen) **yo oigo** | tener (to have) **yo tengo** | venir (to come) **yo vengo** | caer (to fall) **yo caigo** |

# PRESENT PERFECT 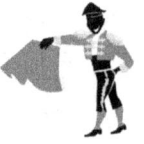 PAST PERFECT

## HABER-auxiliary verb

| Yo | he | había |
| --- | --- | --- |
| Tú | has | habías |
| Él, ella, Usted | ha | había |
| Nosotros | hemos | habíamos |
| Vosotros | habéis | habíais |
| Ellos, Ellas, Ustedes | han | habían |

## PRESENT PERFECT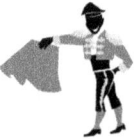

USE HABER + PAST PARTICIPLE (-ado for –ar verbs & -ido for -ir & -er verbs) Example: Juan ha comido. Juan has eaten. Yo he llamado a Juan. I have called Juan. Tú has vivido en México. You have lived in Mexico

## PAST PERFECT

USE HABER + PAST PARTICIPLE (-ado for –ar verbs & -ido for -ir & -er verbs)
Example: Juan había comido. Juan had eaten. Yo había llamado a Juan. I called Juan. Tú habías vivido en México. You had lived in Mexico

# PAST TENSE- PRETERIT & IMPERFECT

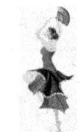

## PRETERIT

| Subject Pronoun | Habl-ar | Com-er | Viv-ir |
|---|---|---|---|
| Yo | Habl-é | Com-í | Viv-í |
| Tú | Habl-aste | Com-iste | Viv-iste |
| Él, ella, Usted | Habl-ó | Com-ió | Viv-ió |
| Nosotros | Habl-amos | Com-imos | Viv-imos |
| Vosotros | Habl-asteis | Com-isteis | Viv-isteis |
| Ellos, ellas, Ustedes | Habl-aron | Com-ieron | Viv-ieron |

OJO take note The preterit tense has two sets of endings: one for –ar verbs and the same for –er & -ir verbs for regular verbs. The nosotros for –ar is the same in the present tense and the preterit tense. Context determines which tense it is referring to. Ex-Hablamos con Juan todos los días- We speak with Juan every day. Ayer hablamos con Juan. We spoke with Juan yesterday.

## PRETERIT IRREGULARS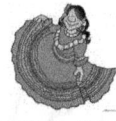

|  | yo | tú | Él, ella, Usted | Nosotros, nosotras | Ellos, ellas, Ustedes |
|---|---|---|---|---|---|
| IR & SER | fui | Fuiste | fue | fuimos | fueron |
| DAR | di | diste | dio | dimos | dieron |
| VER | vi | viste | Vio | vimos | vieron |

Ir and ser have the same preterit conjugation. Context determines which is being used. Ex-Juan fue al cine. Juan went to the movies. Juan fue simpático. Juan was nice.

## U-STEM PRETERIT IRREGULARS

| ESTAR (u-stem) | estuve | estuviste | estuvo | estuvimos | estuvieron |
| --- | --- | --- | --- | --- | --- |
| TENER (u-stem) | tuve | tuviste | tuvo | tuvimos | tuvieron |
| ANDAR (u-stem) | anduve | anduviste | anduvo | anduvimos | anduvieron |
| PONER-(u-stem) | puse | pusiste | puso | pusimos | pusieron |
| SABER (u-stem) | supe | supiste | supo | supimos | supieron |
| PODER (u-stem) | pude | pudiste | pudo | pudimos | pudieron |

## I-STEM PRETERIT IRREGULARS

| HACER (I-stem) | Hice | hiciste | hizo | hicimos | hicieron |
| --- | --- | --- | --- | --- | --- |
| QUERER (I-stem) | quise | quisiste | quiso | quisimos | quisieron |
| VENIR (I-stem) | vine | viniste | vino | vinimos | vinieron |

## J-STEM PRETERIT IRREGULARS

| DECIR | dije | dijiste | dijo | dijimos | dijeron |
| --- | --- | --- | --- | --- | --- |
| TRAER | traje | trajiste | trajo | trajimos | trajeron |
| CONDUCIR | conduje | condujiste | condujo | condujimos | condujeron |

OJO take note The preterit has various irregular verbs. Among them are the : u-stem, i-stem and j-stem. The verbs endings for the i, j and u stem verbs are: -e. -iste, -o, -imos, -isteis and -ieron. There are no accents on any of the preterit -i,-j or –u stems. The –j stems 3rd person plural form is –eron. The 3rd person singular for hacer is hizo.

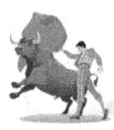

## IMPERFECT

| Subject Pronoun | Habl-ar | Com-er | Viv-ir |
| --- | --- | --- | --- |
| Yo | Habl-aba | Com-ía | Viv-ía |
| Tú | Habl-abas | Com-ías | Viv-ías |
| Él, ella, Usted | Habl-aba | Com-ía | Viv-ía |
| Nosotros | Habl-ábamos | Com-íamos | Viv-íamos |
| Vosotros | Habl-abais | Com-iais | Viv-iais |
| Ellos, ellas, Ustedes | Habl-aban | Com-ían | Viv-ían |

OJO take note: The first & third person conjugations are the same in the imperfect. If the subject or subject pronoun is not listed, context will help you determine subject.

## IRREGULAR IMPERFECT

| Subject Pronoun | Ir | Ser | ver |
|---|---|---|---|
| Yo | iba | era | Veía |
| Tú | ibas | eras | Veías |
| Él, ella, Usted | iba | era | Veía |
| Nosotros | íbamos | eramos | Veíamos |
| Vosotros | ibáis | erais | Veiais |
| Ellos, ellas, Ustedes | iban | eran | Veían |

OJO take note: The imperfect has only 3 irregulars: ir, ser and ver.

## PRETERIT VS IMPERFECT USES

| PRETERIT past completed action with a clear beginning & a clear end. Ex Yesterday I studied. Ayer estudié. | IMPERFECT past repeated action, background action, time, age, whenever you would say 'was' or 'used to' in English Ex Cuando era niño, estudiaba todos los días. When I was a kid, I used to study every day. |
|---|---|
| ACRONYM FOR CHOOSING BETWEEN PRETERIT VS IMPERFECT **SIMBA CHEATED** PRETERIT- **SIMBA** (**S**ingle Action, **I**nterruption, **M**ain Event, **B**eginning Action, **A**rrivals/Departures) IMPERFECT- **CHEATED** (**C**haracteristics, **H**ealth, **E**motion, **A**ge, **T**ime, **E**ndless activities, **D**ate) ||

## FORMAL COMMANDS

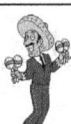

(Formal command have only USTED & USTEDES forms)

Go to the 'yo' form of a verb, drop the –o and add the opposite vowel (-e for –ar verbs & -a for –er and –ir verbs)

| SUBJECT | comprar | vender | escribir |
|---|---|---|---|
| USTED | compr-e | venda | escriba |
| USTEDES | compr-en | vendan | escriban |

**OJO** take note There are 6 irregular Ud/Uds commands: dar - to give: dé, den.

- estar - to be. esté, estén
- haber - to have (auxiliary verb) haya, hayan
- ir - to go. vaya, vayan
- saber - to know. sepa, sepa.
- ser - to be. sea, sean

## THE PRESENT SUBJUNCTIVE

**OJO** To form the present subjunctive: grab the 'yo' form of a verb, drop the –o and add the opposite vowel (-e for –ar verbs & -a for –er and –ir verbs).

| Subject Pronoun | Habl-ar | Com-er | Viv-ir |
|---|---|---|---|
| Yo | Habl-e | Com-a | Viv-a |
| Tú | Habl-es | Com-as | Viv-as |
| Él, ella, Usted | Habl-e | Com-a | Viv-a |
| Nosotros | Habl-emos | Com-amos | Viv-amos |
| Vosotros | Habl-eis | Com-ais | Viv-ais |
| Ellos, ellas, Ustedes | Habl-en | Com-an | Viv-an |

The present subjunctive is used when there are 2 separate clauses in a sentence and used when there is **wish, emotion or doubt ACRONYM: WEDDING.**

example-

WISH: I want Juan to study . Quiero que Juan estudie.

EMOTION: I hope Juan studies. Espero que Juan estudie.

DOUBT: I doubt that Juan will study. Dudo que Juan estudie.

# GLOSSARY OF MEDICAL TERMS

Abscess absceso
Acid Reflux Reflujo esofágico
Acne acné
AIDS SIDA
Alzheimers Disease Enfermedad de Alzheimer
Anemia Anemia
Anesthesia anestesia
Aneurism aneurisma
Angiogram angiografía
Antibiotics antibióticos
anticoagulant anticoagulante
anticholinergic anticolinérgico
anticonvulsant anticonvulsivo
antidepressant antidepresivo
antidiarrheal antidiarreico
antidote antídoto
antifungal antifúngico
antihistamine antihistamínico,antihistamina
anti-inflammatory anti-inflamatorio
antiseptic antiséptico
appendectomy- apendicectomía (Apéndice)
Appendicitis apendicitis
Arrhythmia arritmia
Arthritis (reumatoid) artritis (reumatoide)
attention deficit disorder (ADD) trastorno por déficit de atención

Biopsy biopsía
Bleeding gums sangrado de las encías
Blood clot coágulo sanguineo de sangre
Blood pressure presión arterial
Blood transfusions Transfusión de sangre

Bone density densitometría ósea
Body Mass Index-BMI -IMC-Indice de Masa Corporal
Breast cancer screening Detección de cáncer de seno
breast surgery - Cirugía de mama
Bronchitis bronquitis

Cancer cáncer
carcinoma carcinoma, tumor maligno
cardiac cardíaco
cardiac arrest paro cardíaco, ataque al corazón, paro del corazón
cardiac arrhythmia arritmia cardíaca
cardiologist cardiólogo (a)
cardiology cardiología
cardiomyopathy cardiomiopatía, enfermedad del miocardio
cardiopulmonary cardiopulmonar
cardio-pulmonary resuscitation (CPR) reanimación cardiopulmonar (RCP)
cardiovascular cardiovascular
Cataracts cataratas
Chickenpox – Varicela
Cold catarro
Catheter el cáteter
Cesarean section - Cesárea
Cholesterol el colésterol
Chiropractor quiropráctico
Chronic back pain dolor de espalda crónico
Colonoscopy colonoscopía
Comatose estado comatoso
Common cold catarro
Congenital illness enfermedad congenita
Convulsions convulsiones
CPR reanimación cardiopulmonar

DNR (Do Not Resuscitate) *Orden de no reanimar u ONR*

Dental filling *empaste*
Diabetic Eye Illness Enfermedad diabética del ojo
Dislocation dislocación
Diverticulitis Enfermedad diverticular
Down's syndrome Síndrome de Down
Drainage of tooth el drenaje del diente

emergency exit salida de emergencia
emergency medical personnel personal de emergencias médicas
emergency medical services servicios médicos de emergencia
emergency operations center centro de operaciones para emergencias
emergency operations plan plan de operaciones para emergencias
emergency response respuesta de emergencia
emergency response team equipo de respuesta para emergencia
emergency room (ER) sala de emergencia, urgencias
emergency supply kit equipo de suministros
Epilepsy Epilepsia
Eye Surgery - Cirugía en la vista

FMLA (Family Medical Leave Act) *La ley de licencia familiar y médica*
Fecal blood test *examen de sangre fecal*
Fracture fractura
Fractured bones huesos fracturados

Gall bladder removal - Vesícula biliar (colecistectomía)
Gall bladder stones cálculos biliares
Genital warts verrugas genitales
German measles - Rubéola
Glaucoma glaucoma

Heart Failure Paro cardiaco
Heimlich Maneuver La maniobra Hiemlich
Hemmorroids hemorroides
Hepatitis A/B/C hepatitis A/B/C
Hernia- Reparación de hernia
HIV VIH
Hysterectomy (Partial or Total) ☐-Histerectomía ☐ Parcial ☐ Total ☐
Hyperactive bladder vejiga hiperactiva
Hypertension hipertensión
Hypoglycemia hipoglicemia

Incontinence incontinencia urinaria
Intesive Care cuidados intensivos
Intestal Disease Enfermedad Inflamatoria Intestinal

Joint pain dolor en las articulaciones

Kidney stones cálculos renales

Laparoscopy laparoscopía
Lession lesión

Measles – Sarampión
Menopause menopausía
Menstruation menstruación or período or regla
Migraine Headache Migraña dolor de cabeza
Mumps – Paperas
MRI IRM (Imagen por Resonancia Magnética)

Neonatal neonatología
Neurosurgery neurocirugía
Neurology neurología

Oncology oncología
Osteoporosis osteoporosis
Otolaryngology otorrinolaringología

Pain Management Manejo del dolor
Palpitation palpitación
Peripheral neuropathy neuropatía periférica
Risk factor factor de riesgo

SARS (Severe Acute Respiratory Syndrome) SARS (Síndrome Agudo Respiratorio Severo) Shock choque
Smallpox –Viruela
Stress Test prueba de esfuerzo
Stroke infarto or derrame cerebral

Tachycardia taquicardia
Thyroids tiroides
Tonsillitits - Amigdalectomía
Tube tying –Ligadura de trompas

Ulcers úlceras
Ultrasound ulrasonido

Vaccine vacuna
Vasectomy-☐ Vasectomía
Venereal Disease Infección de transimisión sexual

Warts verrugas

X-Rays Rayos X

# SPANISH TO GO
# For Medical Professionals

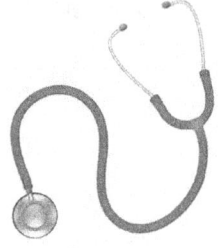

**WORK BOOK WITH PRACTICE EXERCISES & ANSWERS**

Written By:
Georgia Patilis
Illustrations by
Tina Pavlatos

## RECEPTIONIST

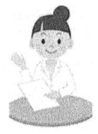

GREETING & GATHERING PATIENT INFORMATION IN SPANISH. You are a medical receptionist.

1) Greet your patient in Spanish. _____
2) Ask for the patient's complete name. _____
3) Ask for the patient's address & telephone number._____
4) Ask for the patient's civil status. _____
5) Ask for your patient's date of birth. _____
6) Ask the patient if he has medical insurance._____
7) Ask the patient for his /her family doctor._____
8) Ask the patient to fill out the form._____
9) Tell the patient that you will be right with him/her._____

PHYSICAL EXAMINATION. INSTRUCTIONS TO PATIENT. You are a doctor. Ask the following questions in Spanish:

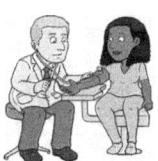

1) How can I help you? _____
2) How do you feel?_____
3) Do you have any discomforts? _____
4) Ask the patient if he has problems chewing or swallowing. _____
5) Ask the patient if he/she has any allergies._____
6) Tell the patient to open his /her mouth. _____
7) Tell the patient o put on this gown _____
8) Tell the patient to breathe deeply. _____
9) Tell the patient to stick out his / tongue._____
10) Tell the patient to relax and sit on the table. _____

## VITAL SIGNS. SIGNOS VITALES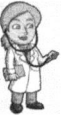

1) Tell the patient that you have to take his pulse and blood pressure and temperature._____

2) Ask the patient how tall he is and how much he weighs.

3) Tell the patient that he has a low grade fever/high fever/ hyperthermia/hypothermia.

4) Tell the patient that he has a fast /slow/irregular / normal pulse.

5) Tell the patient that he has low blood pressure / high blood pressure _____

## MEDICAL HISTORY HISTORIA MEDICA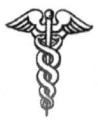

1) Do you have allergies to any food/medicine/antibiotic?

2) Does anyone in your family have heart disease/diabetes/ cancer/stroke/epileptic attacks?

3) Do you drink alcohol / take recreational drugs / smoke?

4) Have you had any surgery?

5) How long have you had these symptoms?

6) Are you pregnant?

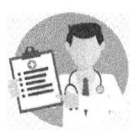

## MEDICAL TESTS ENGLISH TO SPANISH You are a doctor.

1) Tell your patient that he/she needs an X-ray of the lungs, head, and chest.

   _____

2) Tell your patient that he/she needs an ultrasound.

   _____

3) Tell your patient that she needs a pap-smear.

   _____

4) Tell your patient that he/she needs a CAT scan.

   _____

5) Tell your patient that he/she needs a urine analysis.

   _____

6) Tell your patient that she needs a mammogram.

   _____

7) Tell your patient that he/she needs a stress test.

   _____

# First Aid Kit. Botiquín de primeros auxilios. Please pick the correct word from the wordbank.

guantes (desechables o descartables), una mascarilla de reanimación cardiopulmonar, antiinflamatorios, antidiarréicos, jabón desinfectante, crema para picaduras, almohadillas de alcohol, lista de teléfonos de emergencia, aspirina, crema de hidrocortisona, peróxido de hidrógeno, crema para quemaduras, jarabe, yodo, curitas, gasa estéril, bajalenguas, manual de primeros auxilios, esparadrapo, mascarillas desechables o descartables, gotas de colirio-monodósis, jeringas desechables o descartables, venda de gasa, antisépticos, tijeras, antiácidos, pinzas, termómetro, una linterna con baterías de repuesto, algodón, unguento antibiótico, crema para lesiones

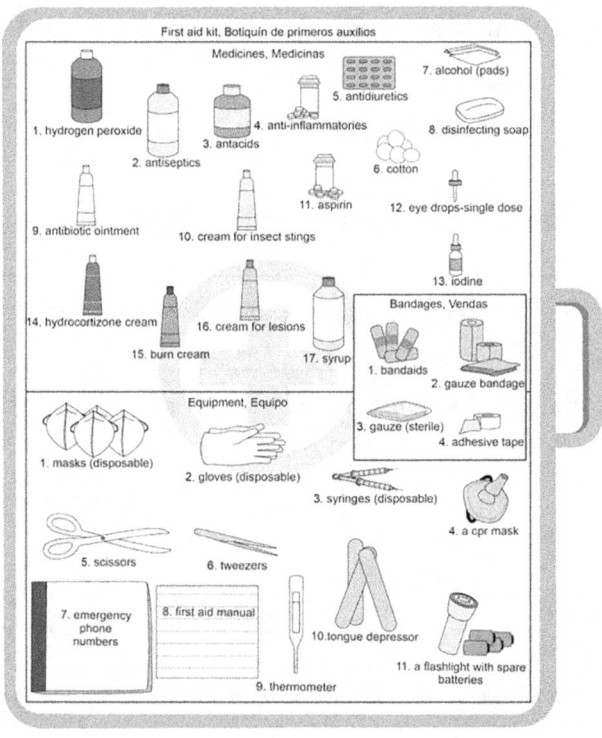

# MEDICATIONS MEDICAMENTOS. Please pick the correct word from the wordbank:

> El inhalador, las gotas para los ojos, el diurético, la cortisona, los analgésicos, la vitamina, el antigripal, los antiácidos, el laxante, el esteroide, la pomada, el supositorio, el jarabe para la tos, los antibióticos, el sedante, el estrógeno, los antisépticos, la penicilina, el descongestionante, el unguento, el antidepresivo, los medicamentos de venta libre, los anithistamínicos, los tranquilizantes/los calmantes, la aspirina, el expectorante, la insulina

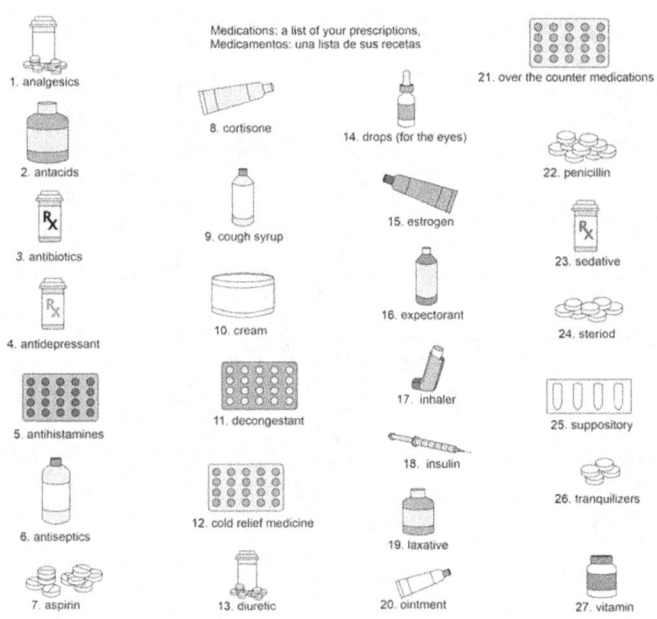

Medications: a list of your prescriptions.
Medicamentos: una lista de sus recetas

1. analgesics
2. antacids
3. antibiotics
4. antidepressant
5. antihistamines
6. antiseptics
7. aspirin
8. cortisone
9. cough syrup
10. cream
11. decongestant
12. cold relief medicine
13. diuretic
14. drops (for the eyes)
15. estrogen
16. expectorant
17. inhaler
18. insulin
19. laxative
20. ointment
21. over the counter medications
22. penicillin
23. sedative
24. steriod
25. suppository
26. tranquilizers
27. vitamin

## UNITS OF MEASURE FOR MEDICATIONS/ STORAGE FOR MEDS. PICK THE CORRECT WORD FROM WORDBANK:

**UNITS OF MEASURE:**
la taza dosificadora, la cuchara dosificadora, la jeringa, las tabletas, la cápsula, el vertidor de medicina, las pastillas, la cucharadita, las bocanadas, la jeringa oral, la botella/el frasco, la cucharada

**STORAGE FOR MEDICATIONS:**
Lejos de la calefacción, en un lugar seco, fuera de la luz del sol, en el refrigerador, al tiempo, lejos del alcance de los niños

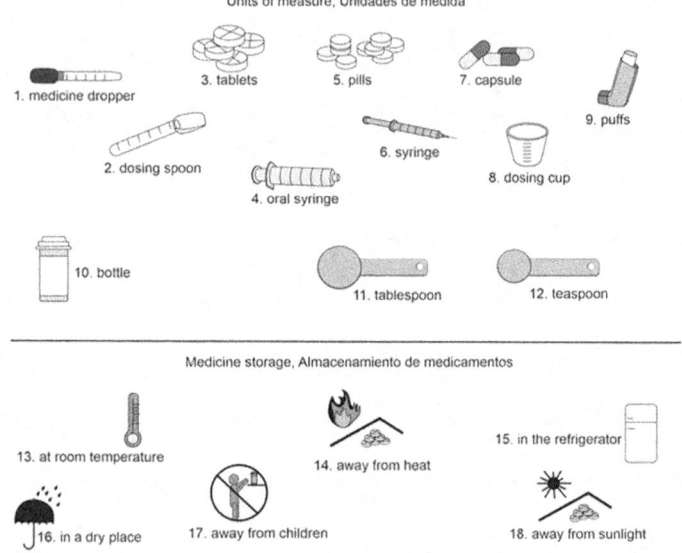

Units of measure, Unidades de medida
1. medicine dropper
2. dosing spoon
3. tablets
4. oral syringe
5. pills
6. syringe
7. capsule
8. dosing cup
9. puffs
10. bottle
11. tablespoon
12. teaspoon

Medicine storage, Almacenamiento de medicamentos
13. at room temperature
14. away from heat
15. in the refrigerator
16. in a dry place
17. away from children
18. away from sunlight

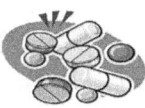 RX Label – La receta Please choose the correct answer for the label in Spanish from the below word bank:

---

El nombre del paciente
Instrucciones al paciente
Cantidad recetada
El nombre del doctor quien hace la receta
El día que llega la receta
Cantidad de rellenos
La fecha de expiración
Nombre y dirección de la farmacia
El número de la receta,
Medicamento, potencia y presentación
El fabricante del medicamento

---

Instructions for medication, Instrucciones para medicamentos

Prescription Label,

3. Name & address of the pharmacy,
2. The name of the prescribing doctor,
4. Number of the prescription,
1. Date of medication,

Jerry's Pharmacy
135 West 81st Street
New York, New York 21007
TELEPHONE NUMBER,
NÚMERO DE TELÉFONO: (555)555-5555
DR K. Vin Nortans
DATE, FECHA: 05/05/22

5. Patient's name,
NO 0060023-08291
ANNA SIMMONS
123 Indiana Ave. New York, NY 11111
TAKE ONE CAPSULE BY MOUTH TWO TIMES A DAY,
TOME UNA CÁPSULA POR BOCA 2 VECES CADA DÍA

6. Medication/strength of the medicine/form of medication,

Take on an empty stomach, 1 hour before or 2-3 hours after eating. Tómese con el estómago vacío,1 hora antes o 2-3 horas después de comer.

CURALLACILLIN 500MG
CAPSULES

7. Prescribed quantity,
QTY 20   MFG XYZ
NO REFILLS, NO SE PERMITEN RELLENOS
You must see a doctor for refill. Usted debe ver a un médico antes de que esta receta pueda ser rellenada.
USE BEFORE, USE ANTES DE:05/05/23
05/05/23

8. Number of refills,

9. Drug manufacturer,   10. Instructions to the patient,   11. Expiration date,

## Pharmacy/Rx Vocabulary

La farmacia por correo, la versión genérica, las recetas de venta libre, la farmacia, los medicamentos con receta, los medicamentos, la receta, el/la farmacéutico/a

## Methods of ingestion

bomba/bombilla, masticar, uso oral, el inyectable, poner gotas, inhaladores nasales, inhalar, inhaladores orales, uso nasal, el inhalador, tragar

## Frecuency

__veces al día, por la mañana, por la tarde, por la noche , cada ___ horas , antes de comer /con cada comida /después de comer, un día sí, un día no, cada tercer día

## How to Take Medication

con mucho agua, no tome con alcohol, en ayunas/ tómeselo con el estómago vacío, no tome leche o productos lácteos mientras esté tomando esta medicina, no lo mastique

## Warnings

Masticar antes de tragar
Manténgase refrigerado
Agítese bien antes de usarlo ,
Necesita tomar toda la medicina
Mantenga los medicamentos fuera del alcance de los niños
Evite exponerse al sol mientras esté tomando la medicina

## Side effects

diarrea, dolor estomacal, mareos, somnolencia, este medicamento puede afectar la capacidad para conducir, boca seca

## Refills /Expiration

esta receta no puede rellenarse, medicamentos caducos, no use después de, fecha de caducidad/fecha de vencimiento, deséchese después de ...esta receta puede_ rellenados

Instructions for medication, Instrucciones para medicamentos

Pharmacy/Rx vocabulary
1. generic version,
2. medications,
3. on-line pharmacy,
4. over-the-counter medications,
5. pharmacist,
6. pharmacy,
7. prescription,
8. prescription drugs,

Method of ingestion,
9. To swallow,
10. To chew,
11. To put drops in eyes,
12. To inhale,
13. Inhaler,
14. Injectable,
15. Nasal use,
16. Nasal inhalers,
17. Oral inhalers,
18. Oral use,
19. Pump,

Frequency,
20. Take this medicine…,
21. ____times a day,
22. Every day…every other day….,
23 very___hours,
24. in the morning/evening,
25. Before eating /with each meal/after eating…, antes de comer/con cada comida/después de comer24.

How to Take Medication,
26. On an empty stomach,
27. With plenty of water,
28. Don't chew; swallow,
29. Don't take with alcohol.
30. Don't drink milk or dairy products while taking this medication.

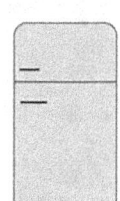

Warnings,
31. Avoid staying in the sun while taking this medicine.
32. Chew pills before swallowing.
33. Keep in a cool place.
34. Keep out of reach of children.
35. Keep refrigerated.
36. Shake well before using.
37. You need to take all of the medicine.

Side effects,
38. This medicine can cause…,
39. diarrhea,
40. dizziness,
41. drowsiness,
42. dry mouth,
43. stomach pain,
44. This medicine can impair driving,

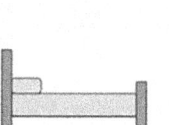

Refills/Expiration,
45. Expired medication,
46. Expiration date,
47. This medicine does not have refills.
48. Throw out after _____,
49. There can be _____ refills.
50. Don't use after _____,

PAIN & BODY PARTS. Choose the correct body part.

_____ 1. Me duelen las orejas.
_____ 2. Me duele la pierna.
_____ 3. Me duele la boca.
_____ 4. Me duele la nariz.
_____ 5. Me duelen los pies.
_____ 6. Me duele la cabeza.
_____ 7. Me duele el pecho
_____ 8. Me duelen las manos.
_____ 9. Me duelen las rodillas.
_____ 10. Me duele el codo.

a. b. c.

d. e. f.

g. h. i.

j. j.

## AILMENTS & SYMPTOMS-DOLENCIAS Y SINTOMAS.

Mix and Match. Please pick the correct English of the Spanish word.

_____ 1. Estoy estreñido

_____ 2. tengo fiebre

_____ 3. Tengo una picadura

_____ 4. tengo una quemadura de sol

_____ 5. Tengo diarrea

_____ 6. Tengo tos

_____ 7. tengo gripe

_____ 8. tengo catarro

_____ 9. tengo vómitos

_____ 10. estoy mareado

A. I am vomiting

B. I am dizzy

C. I have a sunburn

D. I have a cough

E. I have a bee sting

F. I am bloated

G. I have a fever

H. I have the flu

I. I have a cold

J. I have diarrhea

# HOSPITAL FACILITIES & DEPARTMENTS. EL HOSPITAL DEPARTAMENTOS Y AREAS DE APOYO. PICK THE CORRECT WORD FROM WORDBANK:

> **Hospital Departments Los departamentos de un hospital**
> anestesiología, urgencias, cardiología, pediatría, dermatología, otorrinolaringología, oftalmología, hematología, obstetricia y ginecología, Unidad de cuidados intensivos (UCI)/Unidad de vigilancia intensa (UVI), medicina interna, nefrología, traumatología, oncología, gastroenterología, neonatología, neumología
>
> **Hospital Support /Hospital Parts Departamentos de apoyo/partes del hospital**
> El piso número, la sala de espera, la radiología, áreas administrativas, el cuarto del paciente, la admisión, el estacionamiento, la recepción, el consultorio del médico, la entrada, la sala de recuperación, los recursos humanos, la salida, el laboratorio, el directorio, la farmacia

Hospital departments, Departamentos del hospital

The Ward,
1. Anesthesiology,

2. Cardiology,

3. Dermatology,

4. Emergency,

5. Gastroenterology,

6. Hematology,

7. Intensive Care Unit,

8. Internal medicine,

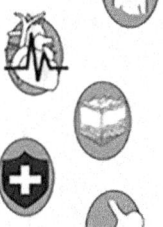
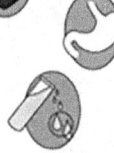
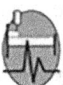
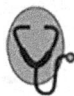

9. Nephrology,

10. Neonatal,

11. Obstetrics & gynecology,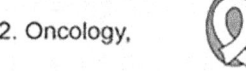

12. Oncology,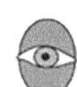

13. Ophthalmology,

14. Otolaryngology,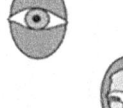

15. Pediatrics,

16. Pulmonary,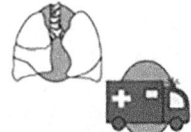

17. Traumatology,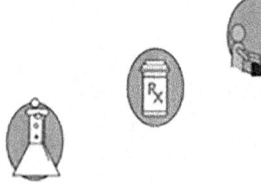

Hospital Support Areas,
18. Administrative offices,
19. Admissions,
20. Doctor's office,
21. Human Resources
22. Laboratory,
23. The pharmacy,
24. Radiology,
25. Recovery,
26. Reception area,
27. Waiting room,

Hospital parts,
28. Directory,
29. Entrance,
30. Exit,
31. Parking,
32. Patient's room,
33. Floor number _____,

# FIRST AID VOCABULARY

## MIX & MATCH

____ 1. low blood sugar          A. puñalada

____ 2. poisoning                B. convulsión/ataque epiléptico

____ 3. gunshot wound            C. pérdida de signos vitales

____ 4. drowning                 D. tos con sangre/vómitos de sangre

____ 5. frost-bite               E. herida de bala

____ 6. animal bites             F. electrocución

____ 7. fractures/bone fractures G. torceduras o esguinces

____ 8. twists or sprains        H. ahogamiento

____ 9. hemorrhages              I. hipoglucemia

___ 10. epileptic seizures		J. mordeduras de animales

___ 11. stabbing wound		K. congelación

___ 12. burns		L. sobredosis de drogas o alcohol

___ 13. loss of vital signs		M. envenenamiento

___ 14. stings (jellyfish or insects)		O. fracturas/huesos quebrados/fracturas de huesos

___ 15. electrocution		P. hemorragias

___ 16. drug/alcohol overdose		Q. picaduras de medusas/insectos

___ 17. choking		R. atragamiento

___ 18. Coughing up blood		S. quemaduras

# FIRST AID PROCEDURES Mix and match

___ 1. Heimlich Maneuver

___ 2. CPR

___ 3. Abdominal thrusts

___ 4. Position of Safety

___ 5. Basic Life Support

___ 6. Mouth To Mouth Rescucitation

___ 7. SAED (Semi-Automatic External Desfibrilllator)

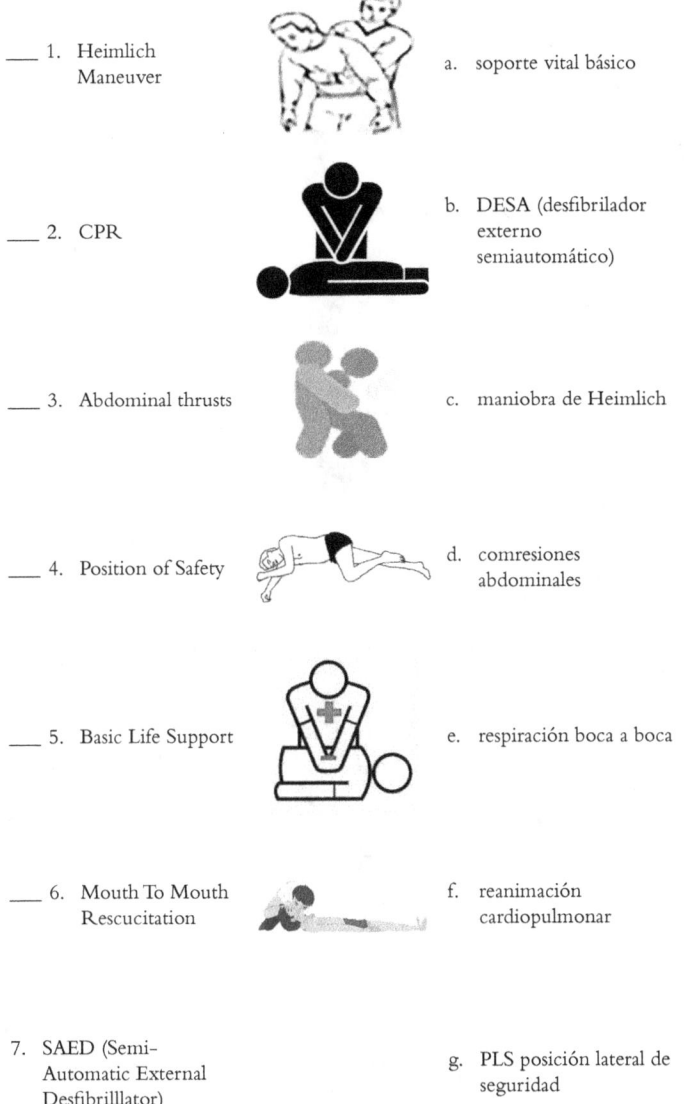

a. soporte vital básico

b. DESA (desfibrilador externo semiautomático)

c. maniobra de Heimlich

d. comresiones abdominales

e. respiración boca a boca

f. reanimación cardiopulmonar

g. PLS posición lateral de seguridad

**Hemorrhages. Hemorragias.** List the 3 types of hemorrhages in Spanish.

1. _____
2. _____
3. _____

Types of hemorrhages, Tipos de hemorragias

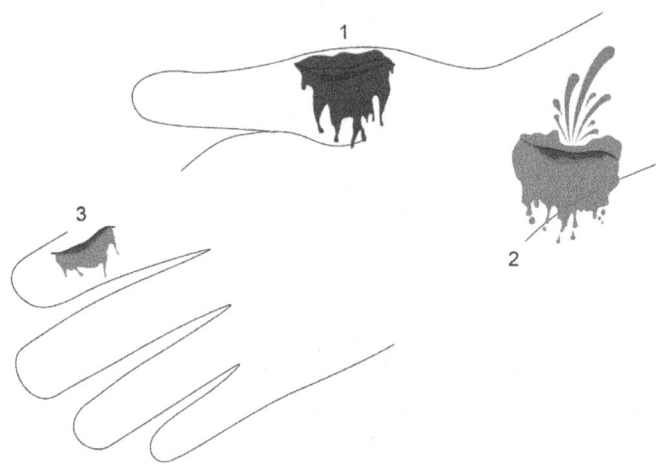

**The wounds–las heridas.** Please label using the word bank.

raspaduras o abrasiones, incisiva/ herida cortante, amputación, herida avulsiva, herida de punción, laceración/ herida lacerada

Wounds, Heridas

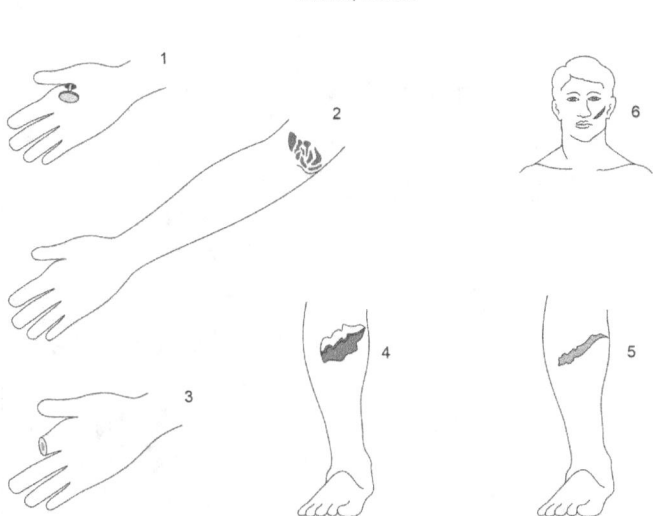

Types of burns–Tipos de quemaduras. Please name the 3 types of burns in Spanish.

1. _____

2. _____

3. _____

Types of burns, Tipos de quemaduras

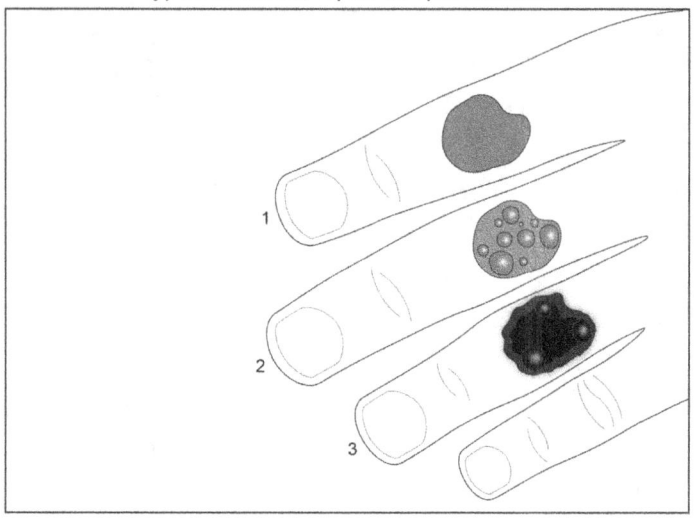

Fractures. Las fracturas. Please label using the word bank.

oblicua, en tallo verde, transversa, compuesta, conminuta, oblicuo desplazado, simple, espiral

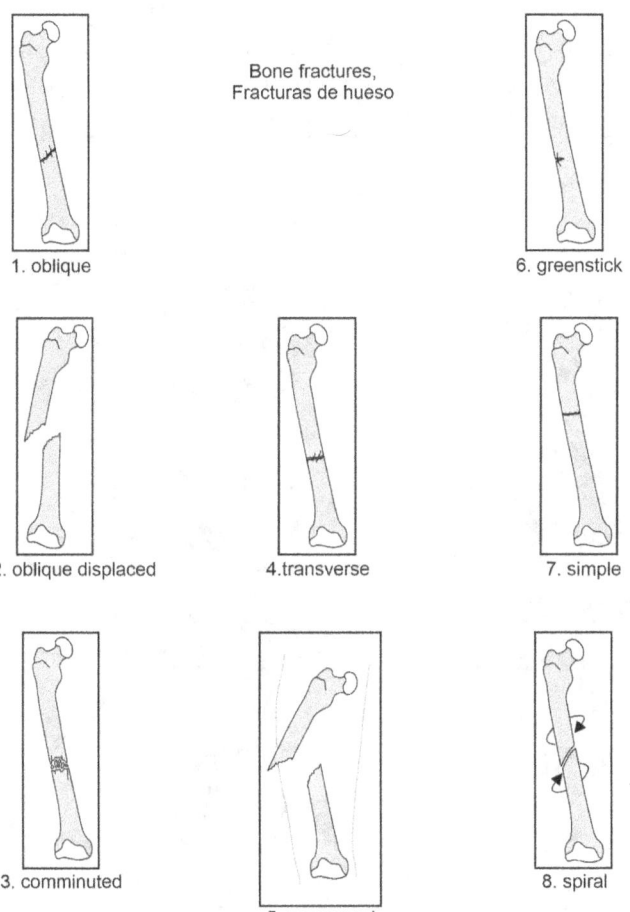

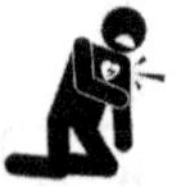

Heart Disease. **Please choose the correct word using the attached word bank.**

> anginas, infarto/derrame, arritmias, acidez, ataque cardíaco, colesterol alto, hipertensión, aneurisma, arteriosclerosis, paro cardiorespiratorio

Heart diseases, Enfermedades cardíacas

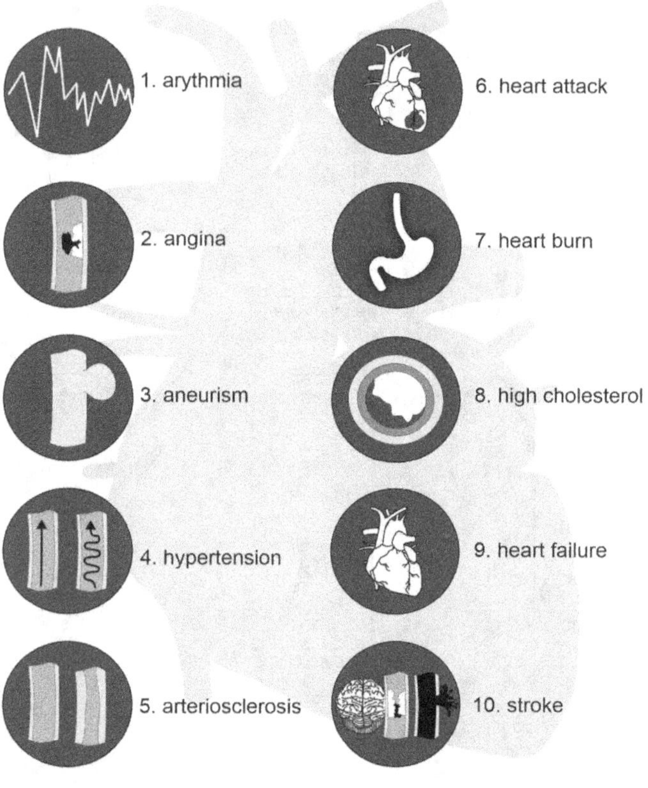

1. arythmia
2. angina
3. aneurism
4. hypertension
5. arteriosclerosis
6. heart attack
7. heart burn
8. high cholesterol
9. heart failure
10. stroke

**La diabetes.** Please match with the correct answer.

_____ polidipsia/ aumento de la sed

_____ poliuira /aumento de la micción

_____ fatiga

_____ visión borrosa

_____ pérdida de peso inesperada

_____ polifagia/ aumento del hambre

_____ llagas de curación lenta

_____ infecciones frecuentes

_____ encías rojas e inflamadas

_____ hormigueo o entumecimiento en las manos o los pies

a. excessive eating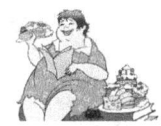

b. wounds that heal slowly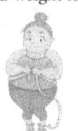

c. increased thirst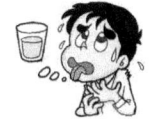

d. unexpected weight loss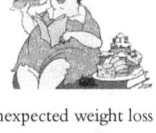

e. frequent infections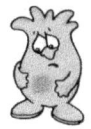

f. excessive/increased urination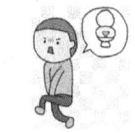

g. red and inflamed gums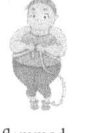

h. fatigue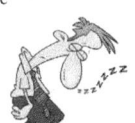

i. numbness or tingling in hands or legs

j. blurry vision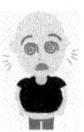

**Diabetes Complications–Complicaciones de la diabetes.** Please choose the correct word from the wordbank.

daño renal, enfermedades cardiovasculares, pie diabético, daño ocular, disfunción sexual, enfermedades bucales, enfermedad vascular periférica, neuropatía diabética

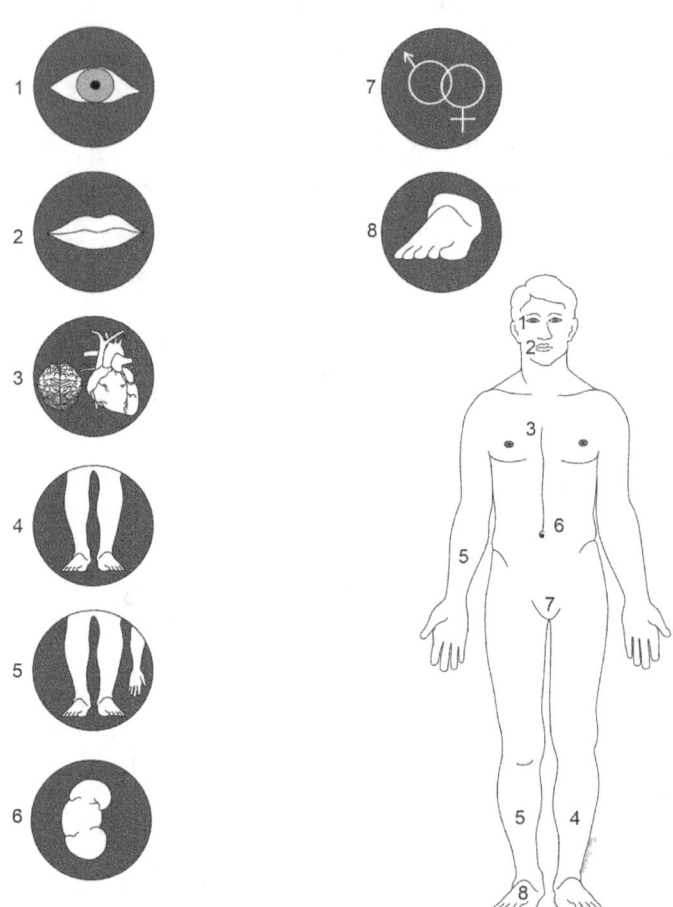

Diabetes complications, Complicaciones de la diabetes

**THE TEETH** Please pick the correct word from the wordbank.

Los incisivos, los molares, el canino, los premolares

## The Teeth, Los dientes

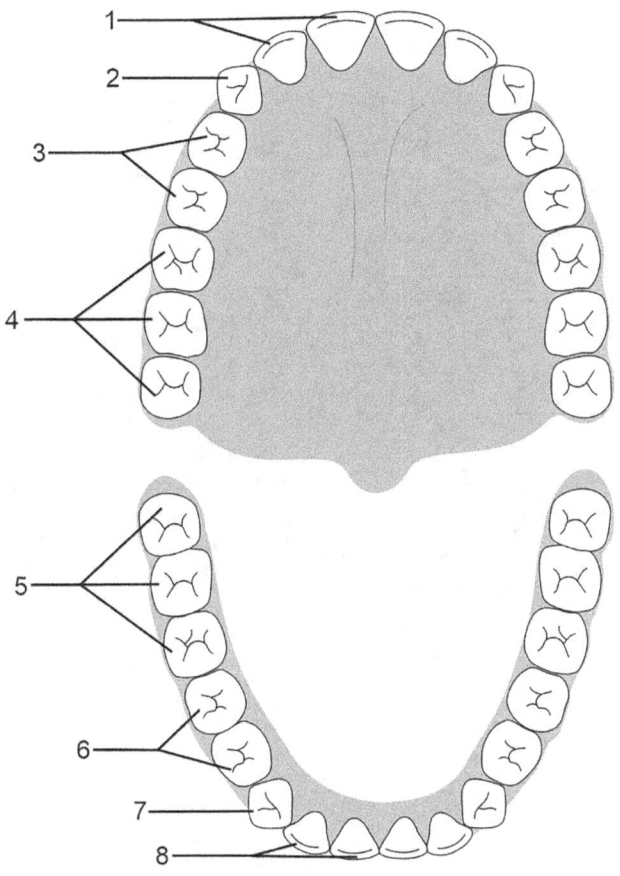

**THE ANATOMY OF THE TOOTH** Please pick the correct word from the wordbank.

El cemento, la corona, la pulpa, raíz, el hueso, la vena, el esmalte, la encía, el nervio, la vena, el cuello, la dentina

## Tooth anatomy, Anatomia del diente

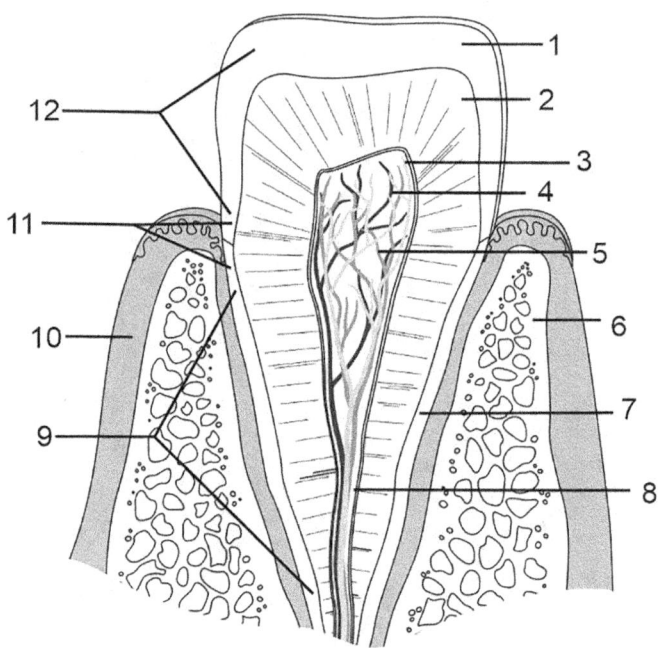

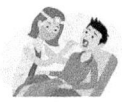

**Los dientes** Match the pictures to the Spanish vocabulary.

A. bleaching  B. dental floss  C. dentures  D. braces

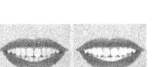 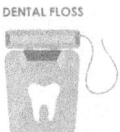 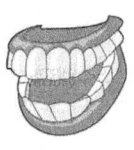 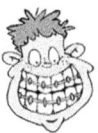

E. halitosis/mad breath  F. crooked teeth  G. periodontitis  H. dry mouth

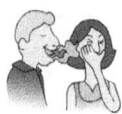 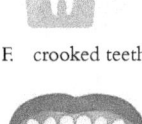 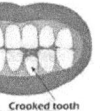 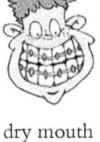

I. swelling  J. loose tooth  K. to gargle  L. to brush your teeth

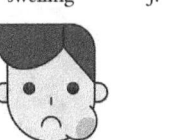 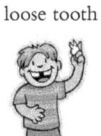 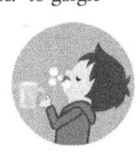 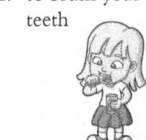

M. retainer  N. baby tooth  O. mouthwash  P. extract a tooth

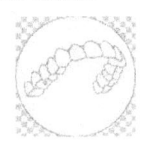 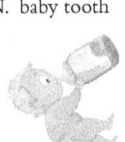 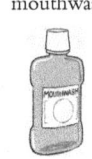 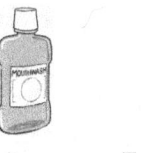 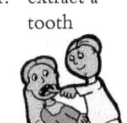

Q. sensitive teeth  R. tooth ache  S. cavity  T. chipped tooth

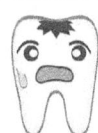 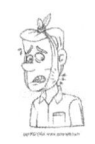 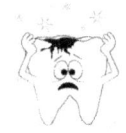 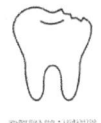

U. root canal/endodontics

_____ 1. enjuague bucal

_____ 2. dientes sensibles

_____ 3. sacarle una muela

_____ 4. diente quebrado

_____ 5. blanqueamiento

_____ 6. hacer gárgaras

_____ 7. periodontitis

_____ 8. halitosis/ el mal aliento crónico

_____ 9. dentadura

_____ 10. endodoncia

_____ 11. cepillarse los dientes

_____ 12. diente flojo

_____ 13. carie

_____ 14. hilo dental

_____ 15. hinchazón

_____ 16. frenos

_____ 17. retenedor

_____ 18. dolor de la muela

_____ 19. diente de la leche

_____ 20. boca seca

**La cabeza.** Please label each part of the head using the word bank.

> el paladar, el pelo/el cabello, los labios, las amígdalas, la pupila, la garganta, el cuero cabelludo, la lengua, el diente, los pómulos, el tabique, el párpado, la pestaña, el seno, la córnea, el mentón/la barbilla, las narices, la fosa nasal, la ceja, el iris

The head, La cabeza

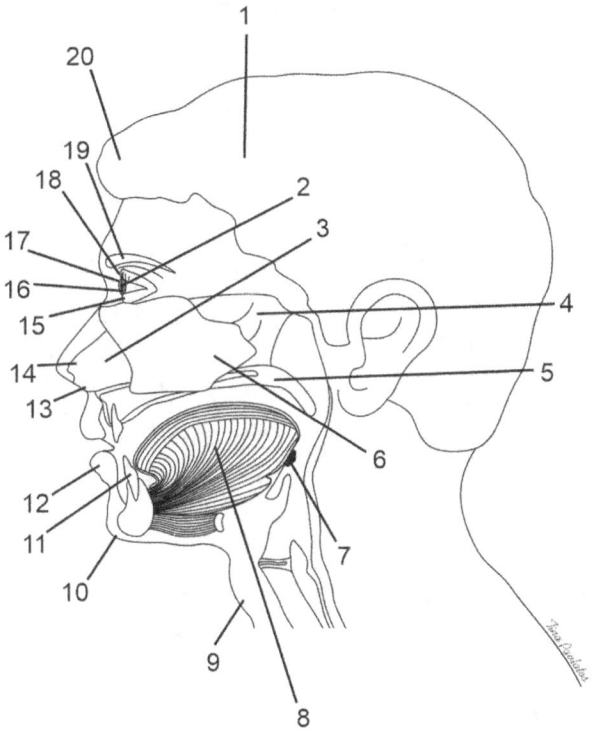

**El ojo.** Please label each part of the eye using the word bank.

lente, coroides, cámara anterior, retina, cornea, pupila, nervio óptico, cuerpo vitreo, fovea centralis, retina central arteria y vena, esclerótica, conjunctiva, cuerpo y músculos ciliares, cámara posterior, iris,

Eye, Ojo

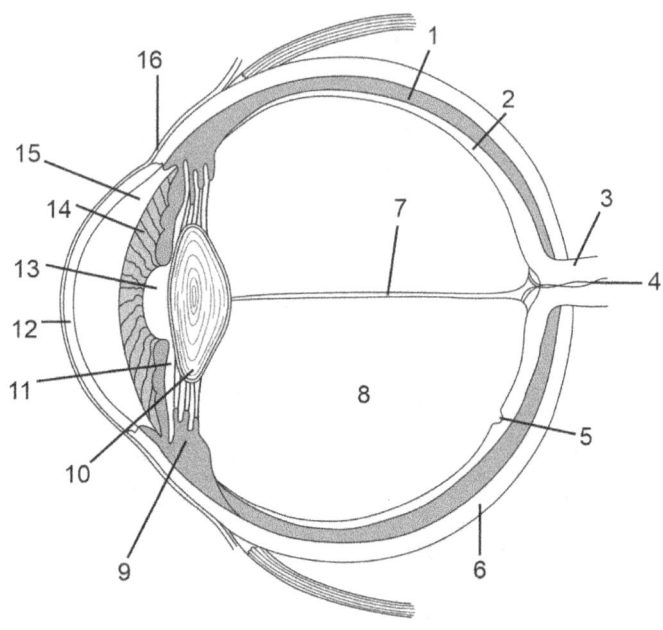

**THE MOUTH-LA BOCA** Please label each part of the mouth using the word bank.

> La lengua, el labio superior, el arco palatofaríngeo, el paladar duro, la úvula, la encía, la amígdala palatina, el freno labial superior, el rafe palatino, el orofaringe, el arco palatoglosal, la encía, el frenillo lingual, el labio inferior, el paladar blando, el frenillo labial inferior, el vestíbulo, los conductos de la glándula submandibular

Mouth, Boca

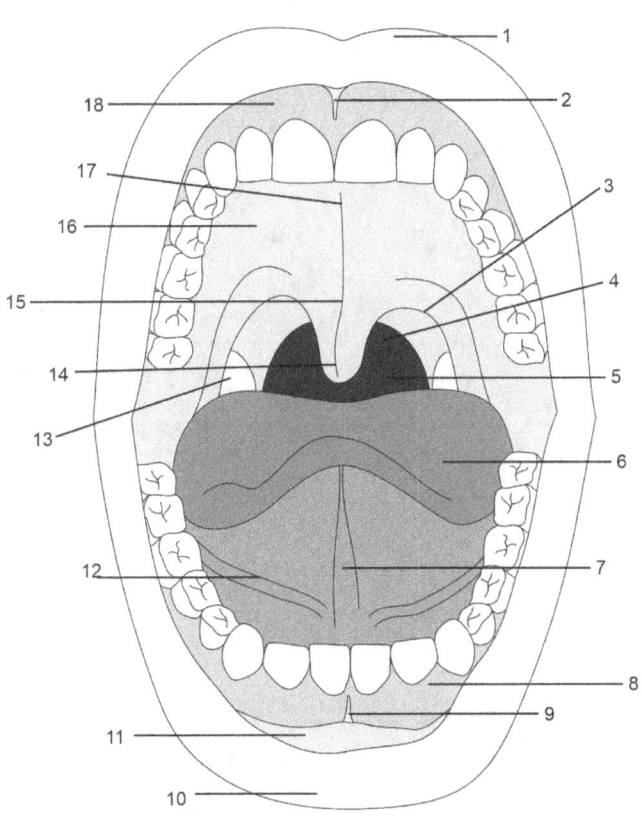

# THE HUMAN BODY-EL CUERPO HUMANO-

Please label the body parts in Spanish using the attached word bank.

> La barbilla/el mentón, la mejilla, la pantorilla, la muñeca, el ombligo, el brazo, el talón, el dedo del pie, el hombro, el dedo, el antebrazo, el codo, el tobillo, la rodilla, el pie, el pecho, el cuello, el pulgar, la boca, la cadera, la cabeza, la oreja, la nariz, los labios, la pierna, la frente, el ojo , el estómago, la palma, el oído, la ceja, la espinilla, la mano

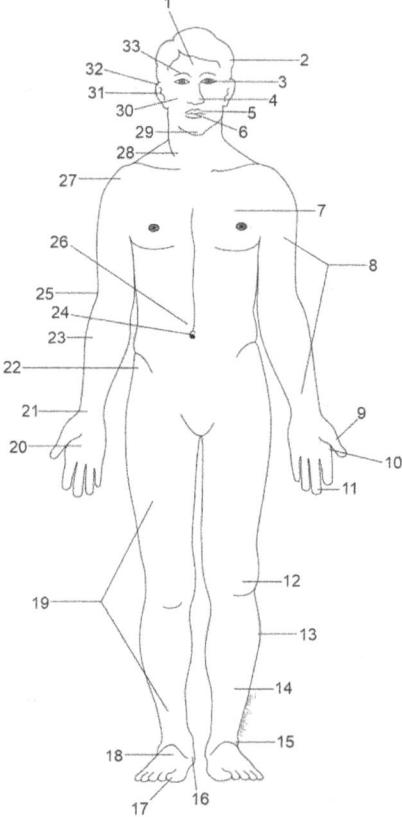

The human body, El cuerpo humano

**The Circulatory System. El sistema circulatorio.
Please pick the correct word from the wordbank.**

vena femoral, arteria femoral, vena cava superior arteria carótida, vena yugular, vena ilíaca, arteria subclavia, el corazón, arteria ilíaca, arteria braquial, vena cava inferior, aorta, vena safena interna, arteria radial, vena subclavia

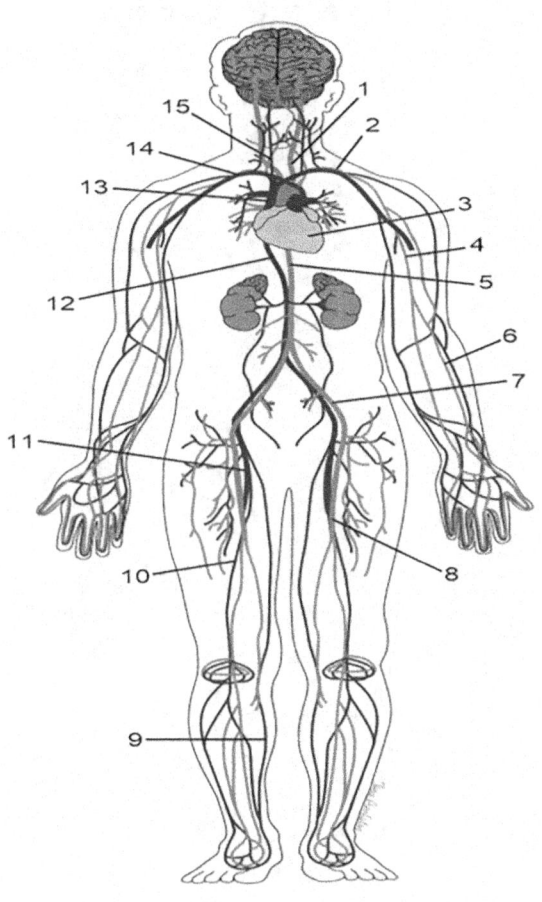

Circulatory system, Sistema circulatorio

**The Heart. El corazón.** Please label the parts of the heart in Spanish using the attached word bank.

aorta descendente, válvulas, arteria aorta, ventrículo izquierdo, vena cava superior, aurícula derecha, vena cava inferior, ventrículo derecho, arteria pulmonaria, aurícula izquierda, venas pulmonares

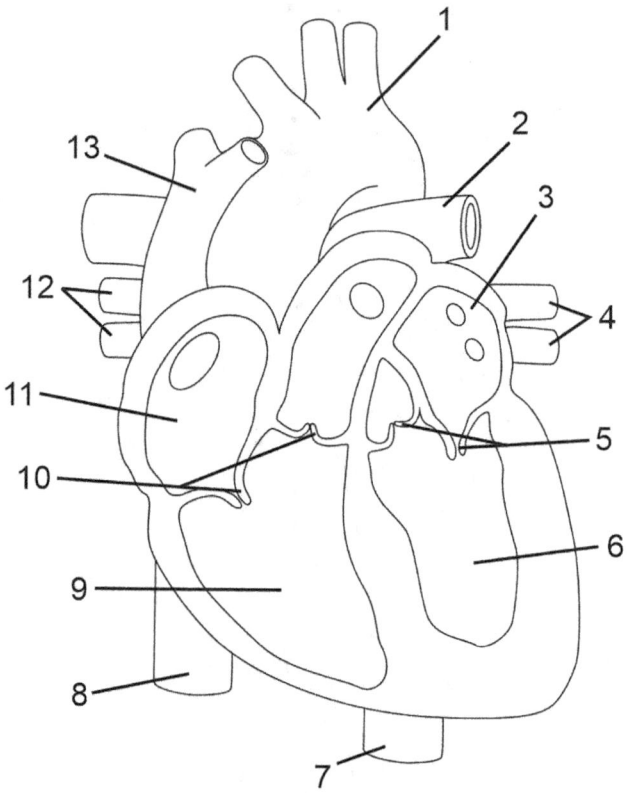

The heart, El corazón

**La mama.** Please label the breast in Spanish using the attached word bank.

---
el pezón, las glándulas mamarias, el tejido conectivo, el tejido graso, los conductos lactíteros

---

## La mama, The breast

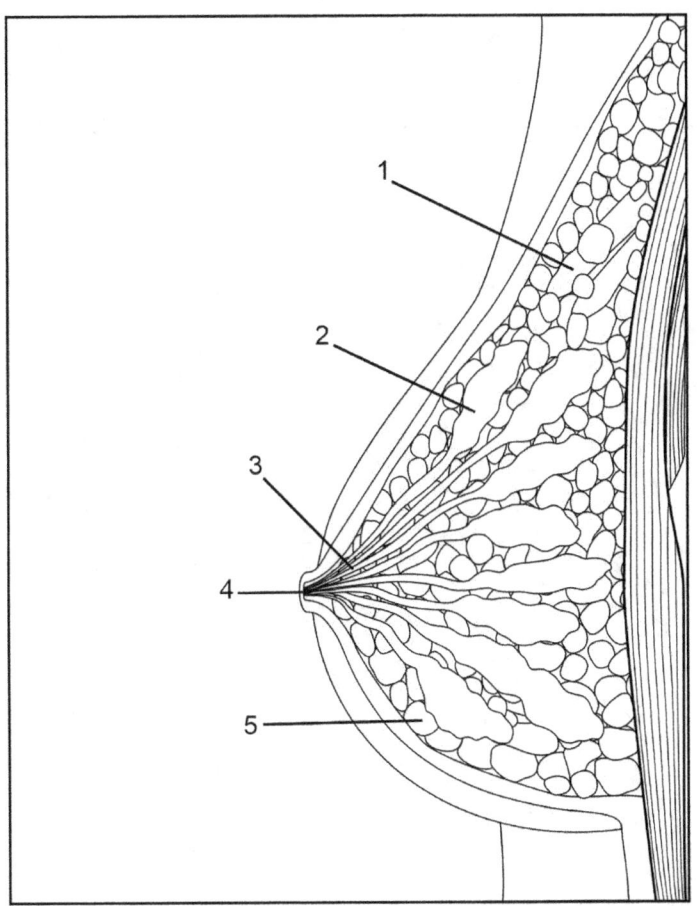

**El Sistema nervioso.** Please label the nervous system in Spanish using the attached word bank.

Nervio tibial, encéfalo, nervio radial, nervio femoral, cerebelo, nervio cubital, médula espinal, nervios intercostales, nervio ciático, nervio peroneo

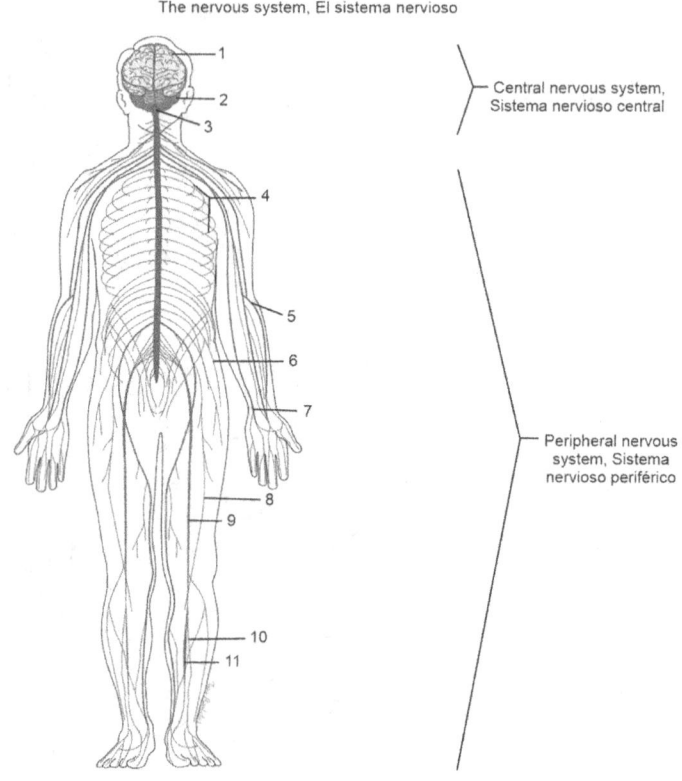

**El aparato digestivo.** Please label the digestive system in Spanish using the attached word bank.

El ano, el hígado, el duodeno, el páncreas, el intestino grueso, las glándulas salivales, el intestino delgado, el conducto biliar, el estómago, el recto, el faringe, la boca, el esófago, la vesícula biliar, el apéndice

Digestive system, Aparato digestivo

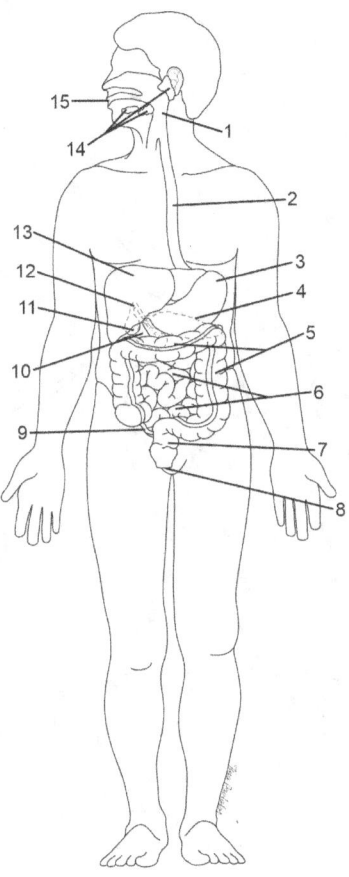

**The Respiratory System. El sistema respiratorio.** Please pick the correct word from the wordbank.

> la fosa nasal, el faringe, las costillas, los centros respiratorios, el diafragma, los bronquios, la tráquea, los músculos intercostales, la cavidad torácica, el pulmón, los bronquiolos, el laringe, la cavidad abdominal, las membranas pleurales

The respiratory system, El sisterna respiratorio

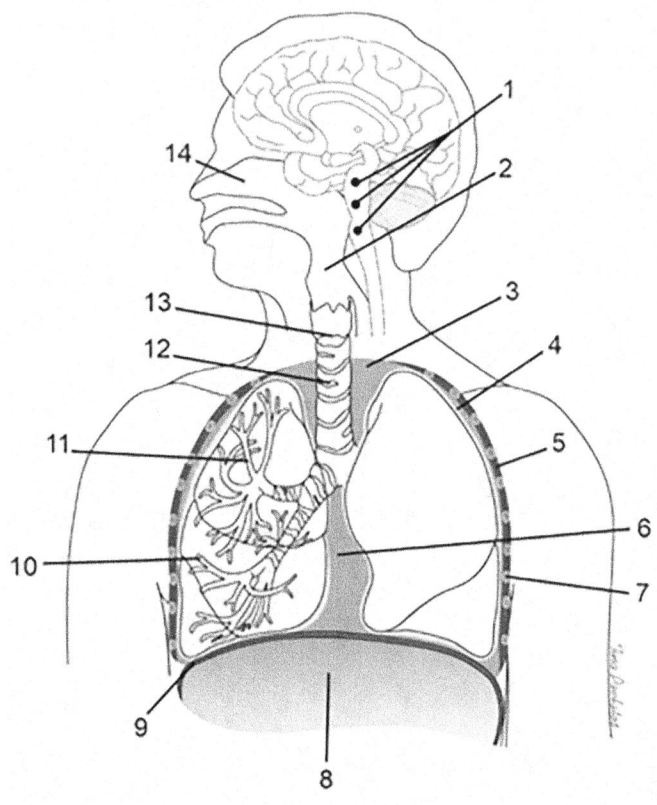

**El Sistema esquelético.** Please label the skeletal system in Spanish using the attached word bank.

Pelvis, metacarpianos, cúbito, metatarsianos, tibia, escápula, radio, tarsales, húmero, peroné, mandíbula, carpos, costillas, rotúla, cráneo, falanges, clavicula, vertebras, fémur, esternón

The skeletal system, El sistema esquelético (el sistema óseo)

**El Sistema reproductor.** Please label the reproductive system in Spanish using the attached word bank.

uretra, útero, vagina, conducto eyaculatorio, pene, testículo, miometrio, glándula prostática, conducto deferente, trompa de falopio, ovario, endometrio, vesícula seminal,

The reproductive system, El sistema reproductor

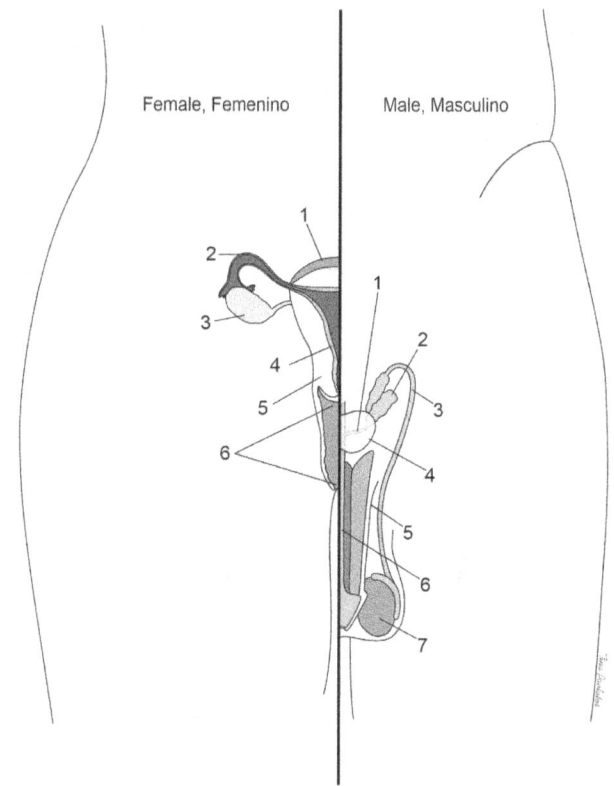

**El Sistema muscular.** Please label the muscular system in Spanish using the attached word bank.

Sartorio, tendón de Aquiles, triceps braquial, gemelos, pectoral mayor, biceps femoral, trapecio, recto del abdomen, masetero, glúteo mayor, esternocleidomastoideo, bíceps, recto femoral, vasto lateral, oblicuo externo

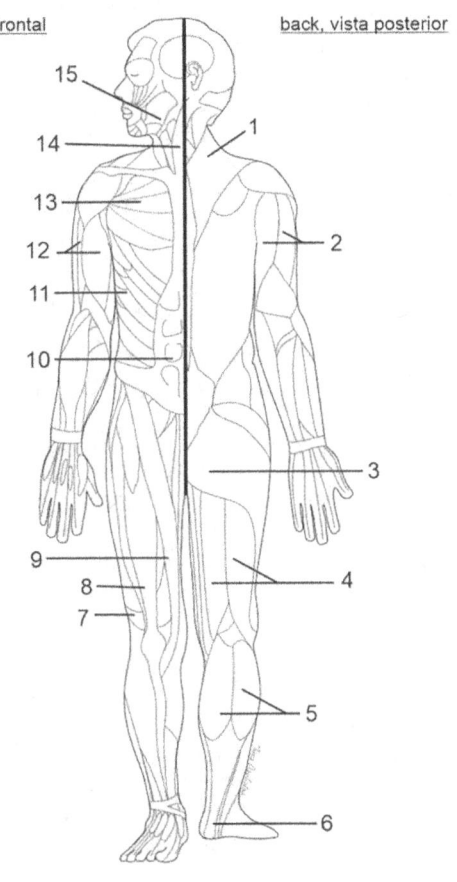

The muscular system, El sistema muscular

**El Sistema endocrino.** Please label the muscular system in Spanish using the attached word bank.

> testículos, glándula timo, glándula pineal, glándula tiroidea, ovarios, el páncreas, hipotálamo, glándulas paratiroides, glándulas suprarrenales, glándula pituitaria

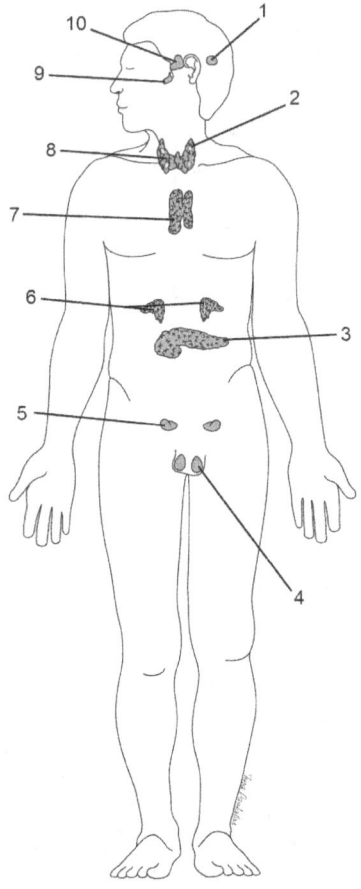

Endocrine system, Sistema endocrino

## GRAMMAR EXERCISES

Greetings. Match the Spanish with the correct English translation.

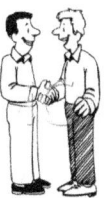

| |  | |  |
|---|---|---|---|
| _____ | Buenos días | A. | And you (formal)? |
| _____ | Buenas tardes | B. | I am from.. |
| _____ | Buenas noches | C. | Thank you |
| _____ | ¿Qué tal? | D. | What is your last name? |
| _____ | Hasta mañana | E. | Where are you from? |
| _____ | Hasta luego | F. | Good morning |
| _____ | ¿Cómo se llama? | G. | How are things? |
| _____ | ¿Cómo está Usted? | H. | My name is… |
| _____ | ¿De dónde es Usted? | I. | Good afternoon |
| _____ | ¿Cómo se siente? | J. | What is your name? |
| _____ | Yo soy de.. | K. | And you (familiar)? |
| _____ | ¿Cuál es su apellido? | L. | How are you? |
| _____ | Yo estoy bien | M. | Good night |
| _____ | Me llamo… | N. | You're welcome |
| _____ | ¿Y tú? | O. | Hello |
| _____ | ¿Y Usted? | P. | See you tomorrow (until tomorrow) |
| _____ | Gracias | Q. | See you later. |
| _____ | De nada | R. | How do you feel? |
| _____ | Hola | S. | I am well |

Question Words. Please choose the correct answer. (1 point each = 10 pts)

1. ¿Por qué? Means..
    a) Who
    b) What
    c) Why
    d) How
2. ¿Cómo? Means...
    a) How
    b) What
    c) Where
    d) Why
    e) Who
3. ¿Dónde? means...
    a) Who
    b) What
    c) How
    d) Where
4. ¿Cuándo? Means...
    a) When
    b) Why
    c) Who
    d) Where
5. ¿Quién/Quiénes? Means...
    a) Why
    b) How
    c) When
    d) Who
6. ¿Qué? means...
    a) Who
    b) What
    c) When
    d) Where
7. ¿Cuánto? means...
    a) Why
    b) When
    c) At what time
    d) How much/many
8. ¿Cuál/Cuáles? means...
    a) How?
    b) Where?
    c) Who?
    d) Which?
9. ¿De dónde? means...
    a) Where (nationality)
    b) What
    c) How
    d) Where (location)
10. ¿A Dónde? means...
    a) Where (nationality)
    b) What
    c) How
    d) Where (destination)

PRESENT TENSE VERBS TABLE. Please fill in the missing conjugations.

| comer | hablar | vivir | tener | ir | ser | estar |
|---|---|---|---|---|---|---|
| Yo como | | | | Yo voy | | Yo estoy |
| | Tú hablas | | Tú tienes | | Tú eres | |
| Él, ella, Ud come | | Él vive | | Él, ella, Ud va | | Él, ella, Ud es |
| | Nosotros hablamos | | Nosotros tenemos | | Nosotros somos | |
| | | Vostotros vivís | | Vosotros váis | | |
| | | | Ellos tienen | | | Ellos están |

PRETERIT. Please fill in the correct conjugations

1. ESTAR
    a) Juan _____
    b) nosotros _____
    c) yo _____

2. QUERER
    a) tú _____
    b) Jamie y yo _____
    c) vosotros _____

3. TRAER
    a) Juan y Jorge _____
    b) nosotros _____
    c) el paciente _____

4. VENIR
    a) tú _____
    b) vosotros _____
    c) ellos _____

5. TENER
    a) tú _____
    b) Jamie y yo _____
    c) yo _____

6. SER
    a) Juan _____
    b) nosotros _____
    c) yo _____

7. IR
    a) Los estudiantes _____
    b) nosotros _____
    c) yo _____

8. PODER
    a) tú _____
    b) yo _____
    c) ellos _____

9. HACER
   a) tú \_\_\_\_\_
   b) nosotros \_\_\_\_\_
   c) ellos \_\_\_\_\_

10. DAR
    a) tú \_\_\_\_\_
    b) yo \_\_\_\_\_
    c) ellos \_\_\_\_\_

IMPERFECT VERB TABLE. Please fill in the missing conjugations.

| comer | hablar | vivir | tener | ir | ser | ver |
|---|---|---|---|---|---|---|
| Yo comía | | | | Yo iba | | Yo veía |
| | Tú hablabas | | Tú tenías | | Tú eras | |
| Él, ella, Ud comía | | Él, ella, Ud vivía | | Él, ella, Ud iba | | Él, ella, Ud veía |
| | Nosotros hablábamos | | Nosotros teníamos | | Nosotros éramos | |
| | | Vostotros vivíais | | Vosotros ibáis | | |
| | | | Ellos, ellas, Uds tenían | | | Ellos veían |

PRETERIT VS IMPERFECT Choose between preterit vs imperfect.

1) 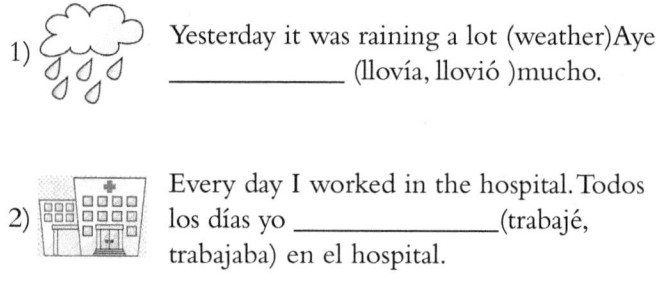 Yesterday it was raining a lot (weather) Ayer _____ (llovía, llovió) mucho.

2) Every day I worked in the hospital. Todos los días yo _____ (trabajé, trabajaba) en el hospital.

3) 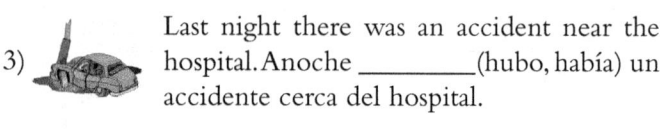 Last night there was an accident near the hospital. Anoche _____ (hubo, había) un accidente cerca del hospital.

4) Juan's car crashed with a truck. El coche de Juan _____ (chocó, chocaba) con un camión (truck).

5) I immediately called 911. Yo inmediatamente _____ (llamé, llamaba) a 911.

6) Juan was unconscious. Juan _____ (estaba, estuvo) insconciente.

7) The ambulance came immediately and they took him to the hospital. La ambulancia _____ (vino, venía) inmediatamente y lo _____ (llevaron, llevaban) al hospital.

8) When I was young, I used to have a lot of car accidents. De joven, _____ (tuve, tenía) muchos choques.

9) Jorge always used to work at the emergency clinic. Jorge siempre _____ (trabajó, trabajaba) en la clínica de emergencia.

11) Yesterday I went to the dentist. Ayer _____ (fui, iba) al dentista.

Ser vs estar. Please choose ser or estar in the following sentences.

1. El hospital _____ (es, está) en Puerto Rico (location)
2. El enfermero _____ (es, está) inteligente y simpático (temperament)
3. El paciente _____ (es, está) enfermo (health)
4. El dolor _____ (es, está) constant (description)
5. Los médicos _____ (son, están) tristes hoy. (mood)
6. Juan _____ (es, está) enfermero (occupation)
7. El estetoscopio _____ (es, está) del Dr. López (possession)
8. La bata (gown) _____ (es, está) es de algodón (cotton) (what something is made of)
9. Yo _____ (soy, estoy) en el laboratorio (location)
10. Nosotros _____ (somos, estamos) aburridos (mood).

# WORKBOOK EXERCISES
# ANSWER KEY

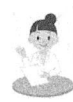

RECEPTIONIST. GREETING & GATHERING PATIENT INFORMATION IN SPANISH. You are a medical receptionist. **ANSWERS WILL VARY.** NOTE: PATIENT SHOULD ALWAYS BE ADDRESSED IN THE USTED FORM, UNLESS HE / SHE REQUESTS OTHERWISE

1) Hola, ¿cómo está Usted?

2) ¿Cómo se llama Usted? ¿Cuál es su nombre y apellido?

3) ¿Cuál es su dirección y número de teléfono?

4) ¿Cuál es su estado civil?

5) ¿Cuál es su fecha de nacimiento?

6) ¿Tiene Usted seguro médico?

7) ¿Quién es su médico primario? ¿Quién es el médico de su familia?

8) Llene la planilla, por favor.

9) Le atiendo en seguida.

PHYSICAL EXAMINATION. DOCTOR GATHERING PATIENT INFORMATION IN SPANISH. You are a doctor. Ask the following questions in Spanish: **ANSWERS WILL VARY.** NOTE: PATIENT SHOULD ALWAYS BE ADDRESSED IN THE USTED FORM, UNLESS HE / SHE REQUESTS OTHERWISE.

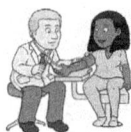

1) ¿Cómo le puedo ayudar?
2) ¿Cómo se siente?
3) ¿Tiene Usted malestar/ molestía?
4) ¿Tiene problemas para masticar / para tragar?
5) ¿Tiene Usted alergías? / ¿Es Usted alérgico/a?
6) Abra la boca, por favor.
7) Póngase la bata, por favor.
8) Respire hondo y profundamente, por favor.
9) Saque la lengua, por favor.
10) Relájese y siéntese sobre la mesa.

VITAL SIGNS. SIGNOS VITALES
**ANSWERS WILL VARY.** NOTE: PATIENT SHOULD ALWAYS BE ADDRESSED IN THE USTED FORM, UNLESS HE / SHE REQUESTS OTHERWISE.

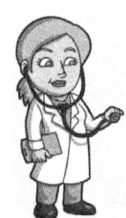

1) Tengo que tomarle el pulso y la temperature.
2) ¿Cuánto pesa? ¿Cuánto mide?
3) Tiene febrícula/ fiebre alta/hipertermia/hipotermia
4) Tiene pulso rápido/lento/irregular/normal.
5) Tiene presión alta/ presión baja.

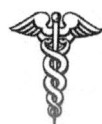

MEDICAL HISTORY HISTORIA MEDICA. **ANSWERS WILL VARY.** NOTE: PATIENT SHOULD ALWAYS BE ADDRESSED IN THE USTED FORM, UNLESS HE / SHE REQUESTS OTHERWISE.

1) ¿Tiene alergias a algún alimento/a alguna medicina/a algún antibiótico?
2) ¿Tiene alguien en su familia enfermedad cardiovascular/diabetes/cáncer/infarto o derrame cerebral/ataques epilépticos?
3) ¿Bebe alcohol? ¿Usa drogas recreativas? ¿Fuma Usted?
4) ¿Ha tenido alguna cirugía?
5) ¿Desde cuándo ha tenido los síntomas?
6) ¿Está embarazada?

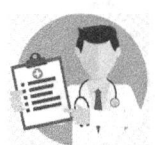

MEDICAL TESTS ENGLISH TO SPANISH You are a doctor. **ANSWERS WILL VARY.** NOTE: PATIENT SHOULD ALWAYS BE ADDRESSED IN THE USTED FORM, UNLESS HE / SHE REQUESTS OTHERWISE.

1) Necesita una radiografía de los pulmones, de la cabeza y del pecho.
2) Necesita un ultrasonido.
3) Necesita un papanicolau.
4) Necesita una tomografía axial computarizada.
5) Necesita un análisis de orina.
6) Necesita una mamografía.
7) Necesita un examen de estrés.

First aid kit, Botiquín de primeros auxilios

## Medicines, Medicinas

1. hydrogen peroxide, peróxido de hidrógeno
2. antiseptics, antisépticos
3. antacids, antiácidos
4. anti-inflammatories, antiinflamatorios
5. antidiuretics, antidiarréicos
6. cotton, algodón
7. alcohol (pads), alcohol (almohadillas de alcohol)
8. disinfecting soap, jabón desinfectante
9. antibiotic ointment, unguento antibiótico
10. cream for insect stings, crema para picaduras
11. aspirin, aspirina
12. eye drops-single dose, gotas de colirio-monodósis
13. iodine, yodo
14. hydrocortizone cream, crema de hidrocortisona
15. burn cream, crema para quemaduras
16. cream for lesions, crema para lesiones
17. syrup, jarabe

## Equipment, Equipo

1. masks (disposable), mascarillas desechables o descartables
2. gloves (disposable), guantes (desechables or descartables)
3. syringes (disposable), jeringas (desechables or descartables)
4. a cpr mask, una mascarilla de reanimación cardiopulmonar
5. scissors, tijeras
6. tweezers, pinzas
7. first aid manual, manual de primeros auxilios
8. emergency phone numbers, lista de teléfonos de emergencia
9. thermometer, termómetro
10. tongue depressor, bajalenguas
11. a flashlight with spare batteries, una linterna con baterías de repuesto

## Bandages, Vendas

1. bandaids, curitas
2. gauze bandage, venda de gasa
3. gauze (sterile), gasa estéril,
4. adhesive tape, esparadrapo,

### Medications: a list of your prescriptions, Medicamentos: una lista de sus recetas

1. analgesics, los analgésicos
2. antacids, los antiácidos
3. antibiotics, los antibióticos
4. antidepressant, el antidepresivo
5. antihistamines, los antihistamínicos
6. antiseptics, los antisépticos
7. aspirin, la aspirina
8. cortisone, la cortisona
9. cough syrup, el jarabe para la tos
10. cream, la pomada
11. decongestant, el descongestionante
12. cold relief medicine, el antigripal
13. diuretic, el diurético

14. drops (for the eyes), las gotas (para los ojos)
15. estrogen, el estrógeno
16. expectorant, el expectorante
17. inhaler, el inhalador
18. insulin, la insulina
19. laxative, el laxante
20. ointment, el ungüento
21. over the counter medications, los medicamentos de venta libre
22. penicillin, la penicilina
23. sedative, el sedante
24. steriod, el esteroide
25. suppository, el supositorio
26. tranquilizers, los tranquilizantes, los calmantes
27. vitamin, la vitamina

### Units of measure, Unidades de medida

1. medicine dropper, vertidor de medicina
2. dosing spoon, cuchara dosificadora
3. tablets, las tabletas
4. oral syringe, la jeringa oral
5. pills, las pastillas
6. syringe, la jeringa
7. capsule, la cápsula
8. dosing cup, la taza dosificadora
9. puffs, las bocanadas
10. bottle, la botella or el frasco
11. tablespoon, la cucharada
12. teaspoon, la cucharadita

### Medicine storage, Almacenamiento de medicamentos

13. at room temperature, al tiempo
14. in a dry place, en un lugar seco
15. away from heat, en un lugar seco
16. away from children, lejos del alcance de los niños
17. in the refrigerator, en el refrigerador
18. away from sunlight, fuera de la luz del sol

### Instructions for medication, Instrucciones para medicamentos

#### Prescription Label, La etiqueta

1. Date of medication, el día que llega la receta
2. The name of the prescribing doctor, el nombre del doctor quien hace la receta
3. Name & address of the pharmacy, nombre y dirección de la farmacia
4. Number of the prescription, el número de la receta
5. Patient's name, el nombre del paciente
6. Medication/strength of the medicine/form of medication, medicamento, potencia y presentación
7. Prescribed quantity, cantidad recetada
8. Number of refills, cantidad de rellenos
9. Drug manufacturer, el fabricante del medicamento
10. Instructions to the patient, instrucciones al paciente
11. Expiration date, la fecha de expiración

## Instructions for medication, Instrucciones para medicamentos

### Pharmacy/Rx vocabulary, La farmacia/ las recetas vocabulario
1. generic version, la versión genérica
2. medications, los medicamentos
3. on-line pharmacy, farmacia por correo
4. over-the-counter medications, la recetas de venta libre
5. pharmacist, el/la farmacéutico,a
6. pharmacy, la farmacia
7. prescription, receta
8. prescription drugs, los medicamentos con receta

### Method of ingestion, Como ingerir
9. To swallow, tragar
10. To chew, masticar
11. To put drops in eyes, poner gotas
12. To inhale, inhalar
13. Inhaler, el inhalador
14. Injectable, el inyectable
15. Nasal use, uso nasal
16. Nasal inhalers, inhaladores nasales
17. Oral inhalers, inhaladores orales
18. Oral use, uso oral
19. Pump, bomba/bombilla

### Frequency, Frecuencia
20. Take this medicine…, Tome estamedicina
21. ____times a day, ____veces al día
22. Every day…every other day……, cada día ….un día sí, un día no, cada tercer día
23. Every___hours, cada ___ horas
24. in the morning/evening, por la mañana/por la noche.
25. Before eating /with each meal/after eating…, antes de comer/con cada comida/ después de comer

How to Take Medication, Instrucciones para tomar la medicación
26. On an empty stomach, en ayunas/ Tómeselo con el estómago vacío
27. With plenty of water, con mucho agua
28. Don't chew; swallow, No lo mastique
29. Don't take with alcohol. No tome con alcohol.
30. Don't drink milk or dairy products while taking this medication. No tome leche o productos lácteos mientras esté tomando esta medicina

Warnings, advertencias
31. Avoid staying in the sun while taking this medicine. Evite exponerse al sol mientras esté tomando la medicina
32. Chew pills before swallowing. Masticar antes de tragar.
33. Keep in a cool place. Consérvese en un lugar fresco y seco
34. Keep out of reach of children. Manténga los medicamentos fuera del alcance de los niños
35. Keep refrigerated. Manténgase refrigerado/a.
36. Shake well before using. Agítese bien antes de usarlo.
37. You need to take all of the medicine. Necesita tomar toda la medicina.

Side effects, efectos secundarios
38. This medicine can cause…, Este medicamento puede causar
39. diarrhea, diarrhea
40. dizziness, mareos
41. drowsiness, somnolencia
42. dry mouth, boca seca
43. stomach pain, dolor estomacal
44. This medicine can impair driving, Este medicamento puede afectar la capacidad para conducir

Refills/Expiration, Rellenos/Fecha de caducidad
45. Expired medication, medicamentos caducos
46. Expiration date, Fecha de caducidad/fecha de vencimiento
47. This medicine does not have refills. Esta receta no puede rellenarse.
48. Throw out after _____, Deséchese después de………
49. There can be _____ refills. Esta receta puede _____ rellenados
50. Don't use after _____, No use después de_____

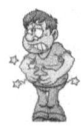

## PAIN & BODY PARTS

| | | |
|---|---|---|
| ____ | 1. | H |
| ____ | 2. | I |
| ____ | 3. | A |
| ____ | 4. | C |
| ____ | 5. | D |
| ____ | 6. | G |
| ____ | 7. | F |
| ____ | 8. | E |
| ____ | 9. | B |
| ____ | 10. | K |

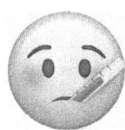

**AILMENTS & SYMPTOMS-DOLENCIAS Y SINTOMAS.** Mix and Match. Please pick the correct English of the Spanish word

| | | | |
|---|---|---|---|
| F | 1. | D. | 6. |
| G. | 2. | H | 7. |
| E. | 3. | I. | 8. |
| C. | 4. | A. | 9. |
| J. | 5. | B. | 10. |

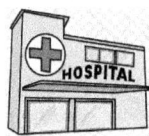

Hospital departments, Departamentos del hospital

The Ward, La sala de
1. Anesthesiology, anestesiología
2. Cardiology, cardiología
3. Dermatology, dermatología
4. Emergency, urgencias
5. Gastroenterology, gastroenterología
6. Hematology, hematología
7. Intensive Care Unit, ICU-(la) Unidad de Cuidados Intensivos (UCI)/(la) Unidad de Vigilancia Intensiva (UVI)
8. Internal medicine, medicina interna
9. Nephrology, nefrología,
10. Neonatal, neonatología
11. Obstetrics & gynecology, obstetricia y ginecología
12. Oncology, oncología
13. Ophthalmology, oftalmología
14. Otolaryngology, otorrinolaringología
15. Pediatrics, pediatría
16. Pulmonary, neumología
17. Traumatology, traumatología

Hospital support areas, áreas de apoyo hospitalario
18. Administrative offices, áreas administrativas
19. Admissions, La admisión
20. Doctor's office, consultorio del médico
21. Human Resources, recursos humanos
22. Laboratory, el laboratorio
23. The pharmacy, la farmacia
24. Radiology, la radiología
25. Recovery, la sala de recuperación
26. Reception area, la recepción
27. Waiting room, la sala de espera

Hospital parts, Las partes del hospital
28. Directory, el directorio
29. Entrance, la entrada
30. Exit, la salida
31. Parking, el estacionamiento
32. Patient's room, el cuarto del paciente
33. Floor number _____, el piso número____

# First Aid Vocabulary

## MIX & MATCH ANSWERS

I____  1. low blood sugar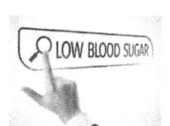

_M__  2. poisoning

__E__  3. gunshot wound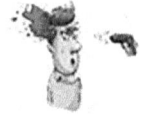

_H___  4. drowning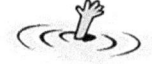

_K___  5. frost-bite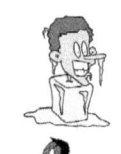

__J__  6. animal bites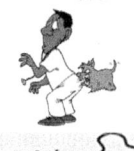

O____  7. fractures/bone fractures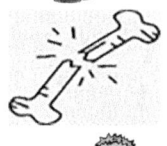

G____  8. twists or sprains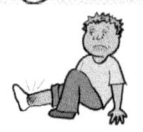

_P____  9. hemorrhages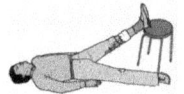

_B_____ 10. epileptic seizures

A_____ 11. stabbing wound

S_____ 12. burns

__C__ 13. loss of vital signs

Q_____ 14. stings (jellyfish or insects)

F_____ 15. electrocution

_L_____ 16. drug/alcohol overdose

_R___ 17. choking

_D___ 18. Coughing up blood

## FIRST AID PROCEDURES ANSWERS

C____ 1. Heimlich Maneuver

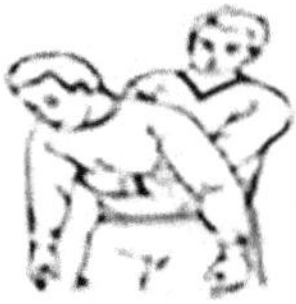

F____ 2. CPR

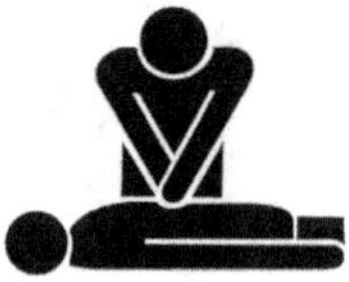

_D___ 3. Abdominal thrusts

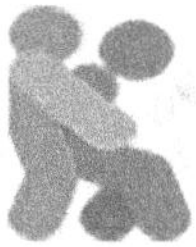

_G___ 4. Position of Safety

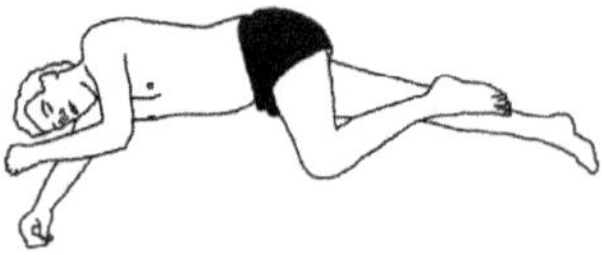

_A___ 5. Basic Life Support

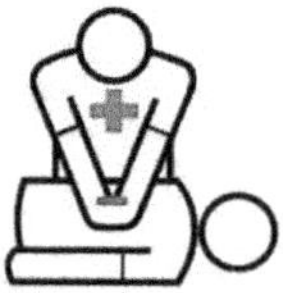

E____ 6. Mouth To Mouth Rescucitation

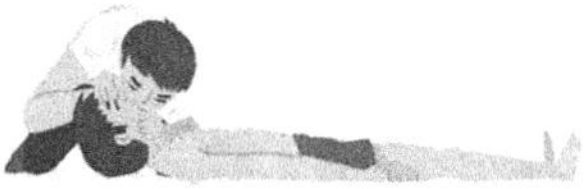

_B___ 7. SAED (Semi-Automatic External Desfibrilllator)

Types of hemorrhages, Tipos de hemorragias

1. venous, venoso
steady, slow flow, flujo lento y constante
dark red color, color rojo oscuro

2. arterial, arterial
flujo pulsante, chorros de sangre,
pulsating flow, spurting blood,
bright red color, color rojo brillante

3. capillary, capilar
slow, even flow, flujo lento y uniforme
bright red color, color rojo brillante

Wounds, Heridas

1. puncture wound, herida de punción
2. scraping/abrasion, raspaduras o abrasiones
3. amputation, amputación
4. avulsion wound, herida avulsiva
5. laceration, laceración/herida lacerada
6. incision, incisiva/herida cortante o incisa

### Types of burns, Tipos de quemaduras

1. first degree burn, quemadura de primer grado
2. second degree burn, quemadura de segundo grado
3. third degree burn, quemadura de tercer grado

### Bone fractures, Fracturas de hueso

1. oblique, oblicua
2. oblique displaced, oblicuo desplazado
3. comminuted, conminuta
4. transverse, transversa
5. compound, compuesta
6. greenstick, en tallo verde
7. simple, simple
8. spiral, espiral

### Heart diseases, Enfermedades cardíacas

1. arythmia, arritmias
2. angina, anginas
3. aneurism, aneurisma
4. hypertension, hipertensión, (high blood pressure), (presión arterial alta)
5. arteriosclerosis, arteroesclerosis
6. heart attack, ataque cardíaco
7. heart burn, acidez
8. high cholesterol, colesterol alto
9. heart failure, paro cardiorespiratorio
10. stroke, infarto/derrame cerebral

**La diabetes.** Please match with the correct answer.

- _C_ polidipsia/ aumento de la sed
- _F_ poliuira /aumento de la micción
- _H_ fatiga
- _J_ visión borrosa
- _D_ pérdida de peso inesperada
- _A_ polifagia/ aumento del hambre
- _B_ llagas de curación lenta
- _E_ infecciones frecuentes
- _G_ encías rojas e inflamadas
- _I_ hormigueo o entumecimiento en las manos o los pies

---

Diabetes complications, Complicaciones de la diabetes

1. eye damage, daño ocular
2. mouth diseases, enfermedades bucales
3. heart diseases, enfermedades cardiovasculares
4. peripheral vascular disease, enfermedad vascular periférica
5. diabetic neuropathy, neuropatía diabética
6. kidney damage, daño renal
7. sexual dysfunction, disfunción sexual,
8. diabetic foot, pie diabético

# Los dientes, The teeth

1. incisivos, incisors
2. canino, canine
3. premolares, premolars
4. molares, molars
5. molares, molars
6. premolares, premolars
7. canino, canine
8. incisivos, incisors

Tooth anatomy, Anatomía del diente

1. enamel, esmalte
2. dentin, dentina
3. vein, vena
4. artery, artería
5. nerve, nervio
6. bone, hueso
7. cementum, cemento
8. pulp, pulpa
9. root, raíz
10. gum, encía
11. neck, cuello
12. crown, corona

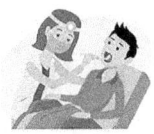

**Los dientes** Match the pictures to the Spanish vocabulary.

| | | | | |
|---|---|---|---|---|
| _____ | 1. O | _____ | 11. L |
| _____ | 2. Q | _____ | 12. J |
| _____ | 3. P | _____ | 13. S |
| _____ | 4. T | _____ | 14. B |
| _____ | 5. A | _____ | 15. I |
| _____ | 6. K | _____ | 16. D |
| _____ | 7. G | _____ | 17. M |
| _____ | 8. E | _____ | 18. R |
| _____ | 9. C | _____ | 19. N |
| _____ | 10. U | _____ | 20. H |

### The head, La cabeza

1. scalp, el cuero cabelludo
2. pupil, la pupila/la niña del ojo
3. nasal cavity, la fosa nasal
4. sinus, el seno
5. palate, el paladar
6. cheekbone, los pómulos
7. tonsils, las amígdalas/las anginas
8. tongue, la lengua
9. throat, la garganta
10. chin, el mentón/la barbilla
11. tooth, el diente
12. lips, los labios
13. nostrils, las narices/las ventanas de la nariz
14. septum, el tabique
15. eyelid, el párpado
16. iris, el iris
17. cornea, la córnea
18. eyelash, la pestaña
19. eyebrow, la ceja
20. hair, el pelo, el cabello

### Eye, Ojo

1. choroid, coroides
2. retina, retina
3. optic nerve, nervo óptico
4. central retinal artery and vein, retina central arteria y vena,
5. fovea centralis, fóvea centralis
6. sclera, esclerótica
7. hyaloid canal, canal hialoideo
8. vitreous body, cuerpo vitreo
9. ciliary body and muscles, cuerpo y músculos ciliares
10. lens, lente
11. posterior chamber, cámara posterior
12. cornea, córnea
13. pupil, pupila
14. iris, iris
15. anterior chamber, cámara anterior
16. conjunctiva, conjuntiva

### Mouth, Boca

1. upper lip, labio superior
2. superior labial frenulum, frenillo labial superior
3. palatoglossal arch, palatoglosal
4. palato pharyngealarch, palatofaríngeo
5. oropharynx, orofaringe
6. tongue, lengua
7. lingual frenulum, frenillo lingual
8. gum, encía
9. labial frenulum, frenillo labia inferior
10. lower lip, labio inferior
11. vestibule, vestíbulo
12. palatine tonsil duct of the sublingual gland, conductos de la glándula submandibular
13. palatine tonsil, amígdala palatina
14. uvula, úvula
15. soft palate, paladar blando
16. hard palate, paladar duro
17. alatine raphe, afe palatino
18. gum, encia

## The human body, El cuerpo humano

1. forehead, la frente
2. head, la cabeza
3. eye, el ojo
4. nose, la naríz
5. lips, los labios
6. mouth, la boca
7. chest, el pecho
8. arm, el brazo
9. thumb, el pulgar
10. hand, l a mano
11. finger, el dedo (el muslo)
12. knee, la rodilla
13. calf, la pantorrilla
14. shin, la espinilla (la canilla)
15. ankle, el tobillo
16. heel, el talón
17. toe, el dedo del pie
18. foot, el pie
19. leg, la pierna
20. palm, la palma
21. wrist, la muñeca
22. hip, la cadera
23. forearm, el antebrazo
24. belly button, el ombligo
25. elbow, el codo
26. stomach, el estómago
27. shoulder, el hombro
28. neck, el cuello
29. chin, la barbilla (el mentón)
30. cheek, la mejilla
31. inner ear, el oído
32. ear, el oído
33. eyebrow, la ceja

# THE CIRCULATORY SYSTEM. EL SISTEMA CIRCULATORIO ANSWER KEY

Circulatory system, Sistema circulatorio

1. carotid artery, arteria carótida
2. subclavian artery, arteria subclavia
3. the heart, el corazón
4. brachial artery, arteria braquial
5. aorta, aorta
6. radial artery, arteria radial
7. iliac artery, arteria ilíaca
8. femoral artery, arteria femoral
9. internal saphenous vein, vena safena interna
10. femoral vein, vena femoral
11. iliac vein, vena ilíaca
12. inferior vena cava, vena cava inferior
13. superior vena cava, vena cava superior
14. subclavian vein, vena subclavia
15. jugular vein, vena yugular

El corazón, The heart

1. arteria aorta, aorta
2. arteria pulmonar, pulmonary artery
3. aurícula izquierda, left atrium
4. venas pulmonares, pulmonary veins
5. válvulas, valves
6. ventrículo izquierdo, left ventricle
7. aorta descendente, descending aorta
8. vena cava inferior, inferior vena cava
9. ventriculo derecho, right ventricle
10. válvulas, valves
11. aurícula derecha, right atrium
12. venas pulmonares, pulmonary veins
13. vena cava superior, superior vena cava

The breast, El seno (la mama)

1. connective tissue, tejido conectivo
2. mammary glands, glándulas mamarias
3. lactation ducts, conductos lactiteros
4. nipple, pezón
5. fatty tissue, tejido graso

The nervous system, El sistema nervioso

Central nervous system, Sistema nervioso central
1. brain, encéfalo
2. cerebellum, cerebelo
3. medulla oblongata, médula espinal

Peripheral nervous system, Sistema nervioso periférico
4. intercostal nerves, nervios intercostales
5. radial nerve, nervio radial
6. femoral nerve, nervio femoral
7. ulnar nerve, nervio cubital
8. sciatic nerve, nervio ciático
9. femoral nerve, nervio femoral
10. peroneal nerve, nervio peroneo
11. tibial nerve, nervio tibial

---

Digestive system, Aparato digestivo

. pharynx, faringe
. esophagus, esófago
. stomach, estómago
. pancreas, páncreas
. large intestine, intestino grueso
. small intestine, intestino delgado
. rectum, recto
. anus, ano

9. appendix, apéndice
10. duodenum, duodeno
11. gall bladder, vesícula biliar
12. bile duct, conducto biliar
13. liver, hígado
14. salivary glands, glándulas salival
15. mouth, boca

## The respiratory system, El sistema respiratorio

respiratory centers, centros respiratorios
pharynx, faringe
thoracic cavity, cavidad torácica
pleural membranes, membranas pleurales
intercostal muscles, músculos intercostales
lung, pulmón
ribs, costillas
abdominal cavity, cavidad abdominal

9. diaphragm, diafragma
10. bronchioles, bronquiolos
11. bronchi, bronquios
12. trachea, tráquea
13. larynx, laringe
14. nasal passage, fosa nasa

## The skeletal system, El sistema esquelético, (el sistema óseo)

1. skull, cráneo
2. mandible, mandíbula
3. clavicle, clavicula
4. sternum, esternón
5. ribs, costillas
6. ulna, cúbito
7. radius, radio
8. metacarpus, metacarpianos
9. femur, fémur
10. tibia, tibia
11. tarsals, tarsales
12. metatarsals, metatarsiano
13. fibula, peroné
14. patella, rótula
15. phalanges, falanges
16. carpals, carpos
17. pelvis, pelvis
18. vertebrae, vertebras
19. humerus, húmero
20. scapula, escápula

## The reproductive system, El sistema reproductor

| Female, Femenino | Male, Masculino |
|---|---|
| . uterus, útero<br>. fallopian tube, trompa de falopio<br>. ovary, ovario<br>. endometrium, endometrio<br>. myometrium, miometrio<br>. vagina, vagina | 1. ejaculatory duct, conducto eyaculatori<br>2. seminal vesicle, vesícula seminal<br>3. vas deferens, conducto deferente<br>4. prostate gland, glándula prostática<br>5. penis, pene<br>6. urethra, uretra<br>7. testicle, testículo |

The muscular system, El sistema muscular

<u>back, vista posterior</u>

1. trapezius, trapecio
2. triceps brachii, tríceps braquial
3. gluteus maximus, glúteo mayor
4. biceps femoris, bíceps femoral
5. gastrocnemius, gemelos
6. Achilles tendon, tendón de Aquiles

<u>front, vista frontal</u>

7. vastus lateralis, vasto lateral
8. rectus femoris, recto femoral
9. sartorius, sartorio
10. rectus abdominis, recto del abdomen
11. external oblique, oblicuo externo
12. biceps, bíceps
13. pectoralis major, pectoral mayor
14. sternocleidomastoid, esternocleidomastoideo
15. masseter, masetero

Endocrine system, Sistema endocrino

1. pineal gland, glándula pineal
2. parathyroid glands (on the posterior surface of the thyroid), glándulas paratiroides (en la superficie posterior de la tiroides)
3. pancreas, páncreas
4. testes in males, testículos en los hombres
5. ovaries in females, ovarios en las mujeres
6. adrenal glands (one on each kidney), glándulas suprarrenales (una en cada riñón)
7. thymus gland, glándula timo
8. thyroid gland, glándula tiroidea
9. pituitary gland, glándula pituitaria
10. hypothalamus, hipotálamo

# GRAMMAR EXERCISES

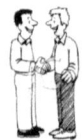

Greetings. Match the Spanish with the correct English translation.

<u>F</u>　Buenos días　　　　<u>B</u>　Yo soy de..

<u>I</u>　Buenas tardes　　　<u>D</u>　¿Cuál es su apellido?

<u>M</u>　Buenas noches　　<u>S</u>　Yo estoy bien

<u>G</u>　¿Qué tal?　　　　　<u>H</u>　Me llamo…

<u>P</u>　Hasta mañana　　　<u>K</u>　¿Y tú?

<u>Q</u>　Hasta luego　　　　<u>A</u>　¿Y Usted?

<u>J</u>　¿Cómo se llama?　　<u>C</u>　Gracias

<u>R</u>　¿Cómo está Usted?　<u>N</u>　De nada

<u>E</u>　¿De dónde es Usted?　<u>O</u>　Hola

<u>R</u>　¿Cómo se siente?

Question Words. Please choose the correct answer. (1 point each = 10 pts)

1. ¿Por qué? Means..
   a) Who
   b) What
   c) Why
   d) How

2. ¿Cómo? Means…
   a) How
   b) What
   c) Where
   d) Why
   e) Who

3. ¿Dónde? means...
   a) Who
   b) What
   c) How
   d) Where

4. ¿Cuándo? Means...
   a) When
   b) Why
   c) Who
   d) Where

5. ¿Quién/Quiénes? Means...
   a) Why
   b) How
   c) When
   d) Who

6. ¿Qué? means...
   a) Who
   b) What
   c) When
   d) Where

7. ¿Cuánto? means...
   a) Why
   b) When
   c) At what time
   d) How much/many

8. ¿Cuál/Cuáles? means...
   a) How?
   b) Where?
   c) Who?
   d) Which?

9. ¿De dónde? means...
   a) Where (nationality)
   b) What
   c) How
   d) Where (location)

10. ¿A Dónde? means...
    a) Where (nationality)
    b) What
    c) How
    d) Where (destination)

PRESENT TENSE VERBS TABLE. Please fill in the missing conjugations.

| comer | hablar | vivir | tener | ir | ser | estar |
|---|---|---|---|---|---|---|
| Yo como | Yo hablo | Yo vivo | Yo tengo | Yo voy | Yo soy | Yo estoy |
| Tú comes | Tú hablas | Tú vives | Tú tienes | Tú vas | Tú eres | Tú estás |
| Él, ella, Ud come | Él, ella, Ud habla | Él vive | Él, ella, Ud tiene | Él, ella, Ud va | Él, ella, Ud es | Él, ella, Ud es |
| Nosotros comemos | Nosotros hablamos | Nosotros vivimos | Nosotros tenemos | Nosotros vamos | Nosotros somos | Nosotros estamos |
| Vosotros coméis | Vosotros habláis | Vostotros vivís | Vosotros tenéis | Vosotros váis | Vosotros sóis | Vosotros estáis |
| Ellos, ellas, Uds comen | Ellos, ellas, Uds hablan | Ellos, ellas, Uds viven | Ellos tienen | Ellos, ellas, Uds van | Ellos, ellas, Uds | Ellos están |

PRETERIT. Please fill in the correct conjugations

12. ESTAR
    a) Juan estuvo
    b) nosotros estuvimos
    c) yo estuve

13. QUERER
    a) tú quisiste
    b) Jamie y yo quisimos
    c) vosotros quisisteis

14. TRAER
    a) Juan y Jorge trajeron
    b) nosotros trajimos
    c) el paciente trajo

15. VENIR
    a) tú viniste
    b) vosotros vinisteis
    c) ellos vinieron

16. TENER
    a) tú tuviste
    b) Jamie y yo tuvimos
    c) yo tuve

17. SER
    a) Juan fue
    b) nosotros fuimos
    c) yo fui

18. IR
    a) Los estudiantes fueron
    b) nosotros fuimos
    c) yo fui

19. PODER
    a) tú pudiste
    b) yo pude
    c) ellos pudieron

20. HACER
    a) tú hiciste
    b) nosotros hicimos
    c) ellos hicieron

21. DAR
    a) tú diste
    b) yo di
    c) ellos dieron

IMPERFECT VERB TABLE. Please fill in the missing conjugations.

| comer | hablar | vivir | tener | ir | ser | ver |
|---|---|---|---|---|---|---|
| Yo comía | Yo hablaba | Yo vivía | Yo tenía | Yo iba | Yo era | Yo veía |
| Tú comías | Tú hablabas | Tú vivías | Tú tenías | Tú ibas | Tú eras | Tú veías |
| Él, ella, Ud comía | Él, ella, Ud hablaba | Él vivía | Él, ella, Ud tenía | Él, ella, Ud iba | Él, ella, Ud era | Él, ella, Ud veía |
| Nosotros comíamos | Nosotros hablábamos | Nosotros vivíamos | Nosotros teníamos | Nosotros íbamos | Nosotros éramos | Nosotros veíamos |
| Vosotros comíais | Vosotros hablabáis | Vostotros vivíais | Vosotros teníais | Vosotros ibáis | Vosotros eráis | Vosotros veíais |
| Ellos, ellas, Uds comían | Ellos, ellas, Uds hablaban | Ellos, ellas, Uds vivían | Ellos, ellas, Uds tenían | Ellos, ellas, Uds iban | Ellos, ellas, Uds eran | Ellos veían |

**PRETERIT VS IMPERFECT** Choose between preterit vs imperfect.

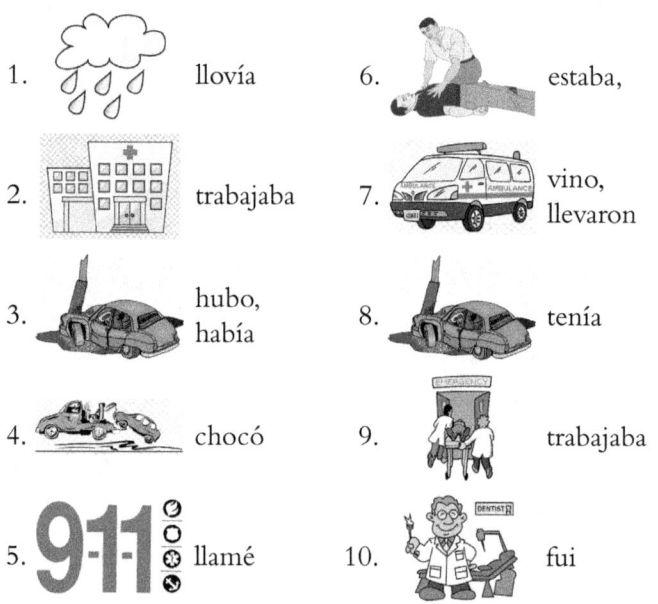

1. llovía
2. trabajaba
3. hubo, había
4. chocó
5. llamé
6. estaba,
7. vino, llevaron
8. tenía
9. trabajaba
10. fui

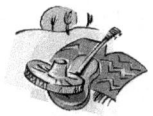

Ser vs estar. Please choose ser or estar in the following sentences.

1. está
2. es
3. está
4. es
5. están
6. es
7. es
8. es
9. estoy
10. estamos

www.ingramcontent.com/pod-product-compliance
Lightning Source LLC
Chambersburg PA
CBHW071402210526
45465CB00001B/214